URETERS

ANATOMY, PHYSIOLOGY AND DISORDERS

RENAL AND UROLOGIC DISORDERS

Additional books in this series can be found on Nova's website
under the Series tab.

Additional e-books in this series can be found on Nova's website
under the e-book tab.

HUMAN ANATOMY AND PHYSIOLOGY

Additional books in this series can be found on Nova's website
under the Series tab.

Additional e-books in this series can be found on Nova's website
under the e-book tab.

URETERS

ANATOMY, PHYSIOLOGY AND DISORDERS

RICHARD A. SANTUCCI
AND
MANG CHEN
EDITORS

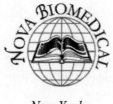

New York

Library of Congress Cataloging-in-Publication Data

ISBN: 978-1-62808-874-8

Library of Congress Control Number: 2013947020

Published by Nova Science Publishers, Inc. † New York

Contents

Preface

The ureters are often overlooked in medical education and real life. We hope to bring to light the importance of ureteral pathology and its management. This book focuses on various types of ureteral diseases including stones, malignancy, and trauma. Management varies from stenting to endoscopic treatment to open and laparoscopic reconstructive surgery. The future lies in improvement of ureteral stents for obstruction, refinement of minimally invasive surgical techniques, and tissue engineered grafts for ureteral substitution.

We want to express our sincere appreciation to the contributing authors in this book. We recognize that clinical work and laboratory research is time intensive. Their dedication to sharing their knowledge echoes the goal of the editors, which is to disseminate medical knowledge to ultimately improve patient care. We also want to thank the staff at Nova publications for their organization and tireless efforts in the making of *Ureters: Anatomy, Physiology, and Disorders*.

In: Ureters: Anatomy, Physiology and Disorders   ISBN: 978-1-62808-874-8
Editors: R. A. Santucci and M. Chen   © 2013 Nova Science Publishers, Inc.

Chapter 1

Ureteral Anatomy and Physiology

Matthew Mutter and Janet Colli
Department of Urology, University of Tennessee, Knoxville, TN, US

Abstract

The ureters are paired muscular tubes with narrow lumen that carry urine from the kidneys to the bladder. This chapter reviews anatomy and physiology of the ureter, followed by a comprehensive analysis of pathological ureteral disorders. Further understanding of ureteral anatomy and ureteral function may lead to the discovery of new pharmacological agents that may be useful in treating ureteral disorders such as facilitating spontaneous stone passage and relieving ureteral colic. In addition, studying etiologies of ureteral pathologies may assist in understanding the disorders which may aide in identifying additional and future treatments.

Anatomy

The ureter is a retroperitoneal, distensible muscular tube that connects the kidney to the bladder and serves as a conduit for urine to flow through. The ureter is positioned in the retroperitoneal cavity with its upper half in the abdominal portion, and the lower half in the pelvis. The ureter commences as an extension of the renal pelvis and crosses posterior to the renal vessels. Next it descends in the retroperitoneal space anterior to the psoas major muscle. It crosses over the bifurcation of the common iliac artery, courses along the lateral wall of the true pelvis, and turns medially to enter the bladder hiatus. In females, at the level of the ischial spine, the ureter lies anterior to the uterine vessels, about two centimeters proximal to the cervix. In males, the vas deferens arches over the distal ureter. The internal diameter of the ureter narrows at three distinct locations: a) at the ureteropelvic junction, b) when it crosses the iliac vessels and c) at the ureterovesical junction. [1]

The ureteral blood supply arises from nearby arteries including renal, gonadal, and vesical; and the ureter is innervated from adjacent hypogastric and renal nerve plexuses. [1]

Physiology

The sympathetic nerves control ureteral contractions by alpha-adrenoceptors cause relaxation by beta-adrenoceptors. Stimulation of muscarinic and adrenergic receptors increases the amplitude of ureteral contractions. [1] In 1977, Tsuchida, et al [2] demonstrated ureteral contractions are originated in pacemaker cells and in 1996 Lammers [3] described the location of these pacemaker cells at the pelvicalyceal border. Kobayashi (4) determined the electrical activity generated propagates in a proximal to distal fashion at an average velocity of 200 mm/second.

Ureteral Disorders

Ureteral Obstruction - Ureteral obstruction is classified as either extrinsic or intrinsic. Extrinsic causes of ureteral obstruction include: retroperitoneal lymphadenopathy, retroperitoneal masses, pelvic malignancies, postoperative complications of pelvic surgery and retroperitoneal fibrosis. Intrinsic causes of ureteral obstruction include: ureteral strictures, ureteropelvic junction obstruction, ureteral stones, radiation fibrosis, infectious causes such as tuberculosis, and ureteral tumors (eg. urothelial carcinoma of ureter). We will provide an overview of the most common conditions affecting the ureter.

Ureteral Strictures - Ureteral strictures are caused by scar tissue, which contracts and reduces the diameter of the ureteral lumen. The narrowed lumen will obstruct the flow of urine and increase the pressure in the collecting system. Acute management of a ureteral stricture involves relieving the obstruction with either a ureteral stent or a percutaneous nephrostomy tube. Long-term treatment options for ureteral strictures include a) endoscopic management, b) open or laparoscopic surgical management. Of importance, Wolf et al [1] found in order for an endoscopic treatment to succeed, the ipsilateral renal unit must have at least 25% function and success rates are better if the stricture is less than 2cm.Initial endoscopic management consists of using a balloon dilator with placement of an indwelling ureteral stent. Another endoscopic treatment of ureteral stricture disease is endoureterotomy, which involves incising the stricture through an ureteroscope [2, 3]. Overall success rates are 50-75% for balloon dilation, and 75-80% for endoscopic incision. There are various techniques for open surgical correction and generally the choice of technique depends on the level of the ureteral stricture, with success rates generally > 90% [4, 5].

Ureteropelvic Junction Obstruction – Strictures of the ureteropelvic junction are caused by intrinsic processes such as congenital ureteral valves or extrinsic processes (e.g. kinking from high insertion or crossing vessels). Intervention of ureteropelvic junction is indicated if nuclear renal scintigraphy demonstrates obstruction in addition to the ipsilateral kidney having function greater than 10%. Treatment of ureteropelvic junction obstruction include: a) endoscopic and surgical reconstruction. Endoscopic correction involves incision of the obstruction (endopyelotomy). [1] If endoscopic treatment fails, ureteropelvic junction reconstruction involves either dismembered or flap pyeloplasty. Open, laparoscopic and robotic surgical techniques have been described. [2]

Ureteral Stones - Calculi may become lodged in the ureter while passing from the kidney to the bladder. Potential sites for ureteral stones to become trapped are: a) where the renal pelvis meets the ureter - the ureteropelvic junction, b) where the ureter crosses the iliac vessels and descents into the pelvic inlet and c) where the ureter enters into the bladder. The degree of renal function impairment depends on whether the ureteral obstruction is partial or complete, is unilateral or bilateral, and on duration of obstruction. Obstruction of the ureter causes acute renal pelvis and ureteral distension which generally leads to renal colic (severe flank pain).

To facilitate passage of ureteral stones, patients can be given alpha-blockers, as ureteral smooth muscle contains alpha receptors. Davenport, et al [1] demonstrated that alpha adrenergic blockade caused a decrease in intra-ureteric pressure, a likely mechanism for increased stone passage when taking

Tamsulosin. Patients who present with stones less than 5mm in diameter are given alpha blockers, and rendered an attempted trial of spontaneous passage.

However, regardless of size, patients who present with infection secondary to an obstructed ureteral stone will require urgent drainage of the collecting system with either a ureteral stent or a percutaneous nephrostomy tube. Ureteroscopy, laser lithotripsy with basket stone extraction can be performed for ureteral stones failing to spontaneously pass.

Vesico-Ureteral Reflux (VUR) - Anatomic structure of the ureterovesical junction is such that under normal circumstance urine is not allowed to flow in a retrograde fashion proximally within the ureter. Although VUR is still incompletely understood, final pathogenesis is related to abnormalities of the intramural ureter. As described by Paquin [1], a 5:1 ratio of intramural ureteral length to ureteral diameter allows urine to remain in the bladder and not reflux from the bladder into the ureter (nonrefluxing ureteral to vesical junction). Treatment of vesico-ureteral reflux consists of ureteral reimplantation at a new bladder location (neoureterocystotomy).

Retroperitoneal Fibrosis - Due to the anatomic location of the ureters, they are susceptible to extrinsic compression. Retroperitoneal fibrosis is an inflammatory reaction that can lead to scar tissue around the ureter and ultimately cause ureteral obstruction. [1] Definitive etiology of retroperitoneal fibrosis can be elucidated in less than thirty percent of cases [2]. Retroperitoneal fibrosis can be treated both medically as well as surgically. Medical management is generally considered first-line therapy and consists of steroids and other anti-inflammatory agents. [3] If medical management fails, surgical treatment is indicated. Surgical management consists of removing the ureters away from the inflamed retroperitoneum (ureterolysis), followed by protection of the ureters by either intraperitonealization or by omental wrapping [4].

Ureteral Trauma/Injuries- The ureters can be subject to injury by external trauma or iatrogenic during surgical procedures. Overall incidence for iatrogenic ureteral injury during abdominal or pelvic surgery is 0.5 to 1 percent [1, 2].

During blunt trauma, the force necessary to sustain ureteral injuries (due to the anatomic location of the ureters) often causes multiple serious co-existing injuries to the patient [3]. The treatment will depend on the mechanism and the location of the injury. If the injury is in the upper ureter, the treatment is to perform an end to end ureteroureterostomy.[4] If the injury is in the mid-ureter, the treatment is either: end to end or trans-ureteroureterostomy, or tubularized anterior bladder flap (Boari).[4] Lastly, if the injury is located in the distal ureter, the best treatment option is ureteral reimplantation.[4] If there is only a partial tear or injury in the ureter, placement of a ureteral stent may be curative in the majority of cases.[5]

Urothelial Carcinoma of Ureter - Urothelial carcinoma of the upper urinary tract is relatively uncommon, accounting for approximately 5% of urothelial carcinoma [1]. The estimated incidence of upper tract urothelial carcinoma in Western countries is about 2 cases per 100,000 inhabitants [2].

Environmental agents are known to lead to the development of urothelial carcinoma [3], with tobacco and occupational exposure the foremost risk factors [4]. Diagnosis can be accomplished with a variety of techniques ranging from the use of imaging in the form of computed tomography to direct visualization during ureteroscopy. The gold standard for treatment is excision with radical nephroureterectomy with a bladder cuff [5]. This surgery can be performed either through open surgical techniques, or more recently by robotic and laparoscopic techniques.

Conclusion

This chapter summarized salient points regarding ureteral anatomy and physiology. In addition, this chapter outlined ureteral disorders and provided a brief overview of treatments of the most prevalent disorders.

References

Anatomy

[1]   Campbell-Walsh Urology, 10th Edition Review, By Alan J. Wein, MD, PhD(hon), Louis R. Kavoussi, MD.

Physiology

[1]   Canda AE, Turna B, Cinar GM, Nazli O. Physiology and pharmacology of the human ureter: basis for current and future treatments. *Urol. Int.* (2007);78(4):289-98.

[2] Tsuchida S, Yamaguchi O: A constant electrical activity of the renal pelvis correlated to ureteral peristalsis. *Tohoku J. Exp. Med.* (1977); 121:133.

[3] Lammers WJEP, Ahmad HR, Arafat K: Spatial and temporal variations in pacemaking and conduction in the isolated renal pelvis. *Am. J. Physiol.* (1996); 270:F567.

[4] Kobayashi M: Conduction velocity in various regions of the ureter. *Tohoku J. Exp. Medicine*, (1964); 83:220.

Strictures

[1] Wolf Jr JS, Elashry OM, Clayman RV: Long-term results of endo-ureterotomy for benign ureteral and ureteroenteric strictures. *J. Urol.* (1997); 158:759.

[2] Netto Jr NR, Ferreira U, Lemos GC, et al: Endourological management of ureteral strictures. *J. Urol.* (1990); 144:631.

[3] Meretyk et al, 1992. Meretyk S, Albala DM, Clayman RV, et al: Endoureterotomy for treatment of ureteral strictures. *J. Urol.* (1992); 147:1502.

[4] Goldfischer ER, Gerber GS: Endoscopic management of ureteral strictures. *Journal of Urology*, 157:770, (1997).

[5] Hafez KS & Wolf JS: Update on minimally invasive management of ureteral strictures. *Journal of Endourology,* 17 (7): 453, (2003).

Ureteropelvic Junction Obstruction

[1] Delvecchio FC, Preminger GM: Technique of endopyelotomy with Acusise cutting balloon. *Braz. J. Urology*, 26:71, (1999).

[2] Gupta M, et al: Open exploration after failed endopyelotomy: a 12 year experience. *Journal of Urology*, 157: 1613, (1997).

Ureteral Stones

[1] Davenport, K; Timoney, A; Keeley, F. Effect of smooth muscle relaxant drugs on proximal human ureteric activity in vivo: a pilot study, *Urological Research*, Volume 35, Number 4, (2007), pp. 207-213(7).

Vesicoureteral Reflux

[1]   Paquin AJ: Ureterovesical anastomosis: the description and evaluation of a technique. *Journal of Urology,* (1959); 82:573.

Retroperitoneal Fibrosis

[1]   Koep L, Zuidema GD: The clinical significance of retroperitoneal fibrosis. *Surgery* (1977); 81:250-257.
[2]   Monev S. Idiopathic retroperitoneal fibrosis: prompt diagnosis preserves organ function. *Cleveland Clinic J. Med*, 62 (2002), pp. 160–166
[3]   Vaglio A., Palmisano A., Corradi D., Salvarani C., Buzio C. Retroperitoneal Fibrosis: Evolving Concepts (2007) *Rheumatic Disease Clinics of North America*, 33 (4) , pp. 803-817.
[4]   Styn NR, Frauman S, Faerber GJ, Wolf JS Jr. University of Michigan surgical experience with ureterolysis for retroperitoneal fibrosis: a comparison of laparoscopic and open surgical approaches. *Urology*. (2011) Feb; 77(2):339-43.

Trauma

[1]   Selzman, A. A. & Spirnak, J. P. Iatrogenic ureteral injuries: a 20-year experience in treating 165 injuries. *Journal of Urology*; 155, 878–881 (1996).
[2]   Elliott SP, McAninch JW. Ureteral injuries: external and iatrogenic. *Urol Clin North Am*. Feb 2006;33(1):55-66.
[3]   Medina D, Lavery R, Ross SE, Livingston DH: Ureteral trauma: preoperative studies neither predict injury nor prevent missed injuries. *J. Am. Coll. Surg.* (1998); 186:641-644.
[4]   Lynch TH, Martínez-Piñeiro L, Plas E, Serafetinides E, Türkeri L, Santucci RA, et al. EAU guidelines on urological trauma. *Eur. Urol.* Jan 2005;47(1):1-15.
[5]   Brandes S, Coburn M, Armenakas N, McAninch J. Diagnosis and management of ureteric injury: an evidence-based analysis. *BJU Int.* Aug 2004;94(3):277-89.

Carcinoma

[1] Petersen, RO. Renal pelvis. LA Biello (Ed.), *Urologic Pathology*, Lippincott, Philadelphia (1986), pp. 181–228.

[2] Oosterlinck W, Solsona E, van der Meijden A, et al; EAU Guidelines on diagnosis and treatment of upper urinary tract transitional cell carcinoma. *European Urol*, 46 (2004), pp. 147–154.

[3] Colin P, Koenig P, Ouzzane A, et al. Environmental factors involved in carcinogenesis of urothelial cell carcinomas of the upper urinary tract. *BJU Int.* 2009; 104:1436–40.

[4] Roupreˆt M, et al. European Guidelines on Upper Tract Urothelial Carcinomas: 2013 Update. *Eur. Urol.* (2013), http://dx.doi.org/10.1016/j.eururo.2013.03.032.

[5] Margulis V, Shariat SF, Matin SF, et al. Outcomes of radical nephroureterectomy: a series from the Upper Tract Urothelial Carcinoma Collaboration. *Cancer* (2009); 115:1224–33.

In: Ureters: Anatomy, Physiology and Disorders ISBN: 978-1-62808-874-8
Editors: R. A. Santucci and M. Chen © 2013 Nova Science Publishers, Inc.

Chapter 2

Traumatic and Iatrogenic Ureteral Injury

Richard A. Santucci[1,] and Mang L. Chen[2]*
[1]Detroit Medical Center, Michigan State College of Medicine,
Detroit, MI, US
[2]University of Pittsburgh, School of Medicine,
University of Pittsburgh Medical Center, Pittsburgh, PA, US

Abstract

Traumatic injury to the ureter is rare. The ureters are elastic and well-positioned in the retroperitoneum to avoid damage. When injured, there is often extensive trauma to other organs. Management of traumatic ureteral injuries is therefore dependent on the management of associated injuries. Iatrogenic injuries to the ureter are more common, especially with the technological advancement in endoscopic, laparoscopic, and robotic surgery. Surgeries most prone to ureteral injury include urologic, gynecologic, and colorectal surgery. Preoperative ureteral stenting is used frequently to minimize risk of injury during non-urologic procedures. However, data suggest that stenting does not decrease ureteral injuries, but may increase their detection when they occur. Management of iatrogenic ureteral injuries is dictated by injury severity and location. Small injuries can be managed with spatulation and primary anastomosis. Distal injuries can be treated with ureteroneocystotomy. Mid and some

* Fax: 313-745-8222, 313-745-4123, E-mail: rsantucc@dmc.org.

proximal ureteral injuries are treated with vesico-psoas hitch or Boari tubularized bladder flap. Transureteroureterostomy can also be used but is frequently avoided. In rare cases of extensive ureteral damage, renal autotransplantation and ileal ureter interposition are considered.

Introduction

Ureteral injuries are uncommon because the ureter is pliable and anatomically well-protected. When associated with trauma, more-urgent associated traumatic injuries take precedence. We make the diagnosis when the patient has been stabilized. Occasionally, the diagnosis is made at the time of exploratory laparotomy. When associated with iatrogenic injury, ureteral damage is often diagnosed intraoperatively and treated simultaneously. Unfortunately, these injuries frequently remain unrecognized until patients present with vague abdominal and flank pain, nausea, vomiting, fever, incontinence, and even renal failure. Some may even lose their ipsilateral kidney if diagnosis is drastically delayed. This chapter reviews relevant ureteric anatomy, etiology, diagnosis, and management of ureteral injuries.

Anatomy

The ureter is a tubular retroperitoneal structure that transports urine made in the kidney into the bladder. It is divided into 3 segments: the proximal, mid, and distal ureter. The proximal ureter starts at the ureteropelvic junction and ends at the level of the sacroiliac joint. The left proximal ureter is posterior to the body of the pancreas and duodenal-jejunal junction. The right is behind the 2nd portion of the duodenum. The mid ureters course behind the gonadal veins and colonic mesenteries and terminate just as they cross over the bifurcation of the common iliac arteries. The distal ureters in men pass behind the vas deferens prior to entering the bladder. In women, the distal ureters pass behind the broad ligament and uterine artery. They are close to the cervix prior to reaching the bladder.

The ureteral blood supply comes from multiple sources. The medial ureteric vasculature generally originates from the renal arteries, aorta, gonadal arteries, and iliac arteries. The lateral arterial sources are the vesical, uterine, and middle rectal arteries. These small ureteric arteries lie in the adventitia and course longitudinally, anastomosing extensively to one another.

Lymphatic drainage from the ureters occurs regionally. For example, the distal and mid ureter drains to the external, internal, and common iliac lymph nodes.

Etiology

Due to the elasticity and retroperitoneal location of the ureter, it is rarely injured in trauma. Less than 1% of all genitourinary trauma involves the ureter [1]. Penetrating trauma, such as gunshot and stab wounds, damages the ureter more often than blunt trauma like motor vehicle accidents. Elliott and McAninch reviewed their traumatic ureteral injury results over a 25-year period and found that the upper ureters were the most common site of injury, with 27 proximal injuries out of 38 involved ureters (70%), followed by distal ureters in 8 (22%) and mid ureters in 3 (8%) [1]. However, Best et al found that proximal upper ureteral injuries occurred in 15 of 57 patients (26%), mid in 21 (37%), and distal in 21 (37%) [2]. Both long term studies confirm that gunshot wounds are, by far, the most common cause of ureteral injury in the United States. They account for over 90% of ureteral injuries, followed by stab wounds (5%), and blunt trauma (4%) [1]. For gunshot wounds to the lower urinary tract, ureteral injuries occur in about 20% of patients (often concomitant with bladder or gastrointestinal injury), and isolated ureteral injuries occur more often when bullets have a lower abdominal entry with an anteroposterior trajectory [3].

Blunt trauma, especially those associated with rapid acceleration-deceleration, can cause proximal or distal ureteral injury at its connection with the renal pelvis and bladder. Proximal ureter or ureteropelvic junction (UPJ) injuries occur less frequently than other blunt trauma ureteral injuries [4]. UPJ disruptions tend to be on the right side, and they occur more often in children [5]. Patients with collection system obstruction, such as ureteropelvic junction narrowing with associated hydronephrosis, may develop injury from even minor trauma [6].

Iatrogenic ureteral injuries are much more common than external traumatic injuries, accounting for 75% of all ureteral injuries [7]. Gynecologic surgeries account for most (73%), followed by general surgery (14%) and urologic (14%) procedures [7]. Increased use of laparoscopic and robotic surgery has also increased the risk of ureteral injuries [8-10]. Other surgical procedures known for potential ureteral complications include colorectal, vascular, and spinal surgery.

Gynecologic procedures are traditionally associated with ureteral injury given the proximity of the uterine vessels to the ureter. Ureteral injuries occur in 1.3-2.2% of these procedures [11]. Laparoscopic hysterectomies lead to more ureteral injuries than open procedures [11]. Vaginal hysterectomies rarely cause ureteral injury (0.03%), but they do cause more bladder injuries [12]. In addition, intraoperative injuries are frequently missed. Most cases are diagnosed 2-4 weeks postoperatively when the patient develops flank pain. The delayed presentation suggests thermal or cautery injury with tissue ischemia and resultant urinary extravasation or obstruction occurring later. As a result, gynecologists sometimes perform a post-hysterectomy cystoscopy to determine whether a ureteral jet can be identified from both ureteral orifices. Risk factors for ureteral injury include novice laparoscopic/robotic surgeon, prior pelvic surgery, prior radiation, inflammatory processes like endometriosis and diverticulitis, pelvic organ prolapse, and a large uterus.

Other pelvic surgeries that lead to iatrogenic ureteral damage include abdominal perineal resections and low anterior resections for rectal and colon cancer. The left ureter is more commonly injured than the right given its proximity to the sigmoid mesentery. The incidence of injury is 0.3-5.7% [13]. More ureteral injuries occurred with laparoscopic procedures than with open surgery [14].

Retroperitoneal vascular surgery and lymphadenectomy can also cause ureteral injury. The overall incidence is 2-4% [13]. Extrinsic compression and local inflammation from vascular aneurysms, prior radiation, vascular graft infections, and other fibrotic processes increase the risk of ureteral involvement during and after surgery.

About 20% of patients have asymptomatic hydronephrosis after vascular surgery; most ureteric obstruction resolves spontaneously within 2-3 months. One of the most devastating ureteral injuries is delayed development of an uretero-vascular fistula (Figure 1). Brisk bleeding and voluminous hematuria can occur in these situations. A high index of suspicion is required for diagnosis and prompt action can prevent death. Risk factors for fistula development are anterior graft placement, chronic ureteral stenting, and obstruction.

Urologists, especially those performing ureteroscopic procedures, also cause iatrogenic ureteral injuries [15]. Advances in endoscopic, fiber optic, and laser technology lowered the incidence of injury from 42% to 14% over the past decade. Types of injuries include ureteral stricture, perforation, avulsion, and submucosal tunneling.

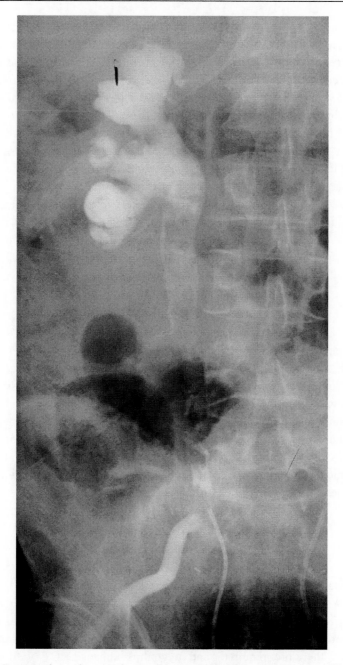

Figure 1. Retrograde pyelogram demonstrates opacification of the external iliac artery, confirming the presence of an uretero-vascular fistula. This patient had profuse gross hematuria.

Risk factors include novice endoscopist, stone impaction, prior radiation or instrumentation, and quality of available equipment such as a lubriciously coated wire, up-to-date laser technology, and a well-maintained and modern flexible ureteroscope. The use of ureteral access sheaths can also increase risk of ureteral wall injury, especially in patients not treated with double-J stenting prior to using the access sheaths [16]. Other urologic procedures that can lead to ureteral injury include radical prostatectomies, retroperitoneal lymph node dissections (RPLNDs), partial nephrectomies, and cystectomies. Similar to other pelvic or retroperitoneal surgeries, unrecognized thermal injuries can lead to delayed urinary tract obstruction or extravasation.

Radiation and chemotherapy rarely lead to ureteral injury, but retroperitoneal fibrosis from radiation-induced inflammation, direct radiation damage to ureteral tissue, and a desmoplastic reaction secondary to chemotherapy can cause urinary tract obstruction.

Clinical Presentation

For unrecognized iatrogenic ureteral injuries, patients can present with flank pain, fever, incontinence from a fistula, ileus from peritoneal urinary extravasation, abscess, and hematuria. Some present without any symptoms and are found later to have hydronephrosis, renal parenchymal thinning, and loss of kidney function. Physical exam can occasionally reveal a distended or tender abdomen, costovertebral angle tenderness to percussion, flank ecchymosis, or fluid drainage from an abdominal or vaginal wound. Traumatic ureteral injury symptoms are frequently and purposefully not elicited due to their frequent association with life threatening non-urologic injuries.

Diagnosis and Evaluation

Physical exam is inadequate for diagnosis and evaluation of ureteral injuries. A high index of suspicion is required. Useful laboratory studies include urinalysis and serum creatinine. Hematuria is seen in 74% of ureteral injuries, indicating that lack of hematuria does not rule out ureteral injury [1]. Imaging is therefore required, and a contrast-enhanced CT with delayed imaging is the modality of choice. Contrast extravasation near the renal pelvis is suggestive of renal pelvis or proximal ureteral injury; contrast elsewhere in the retroperitoneum has a less predictable location of injury.

In a stable patient with a suspected ureteral injury as determined by a urologic workup, cystoscopy with retrograde pyelography is the best way to confirm and locate the injury (Figure 2). One can also place a temporizing and sometimes therapeutic ureteral stent concomitantly.

Studies that are not often used include magnetic resonance imaging (MRI) and intravenous pyelography (IVP). MRI is frequently inappropriate in the acute setting, but MR urography has been introduced as an alternative to CT to avoid ionizing radiation and iodine contrast dye allergies [17]. IVP may have a role in the non-imaged patient requiring emergent exploratory laparotomy with suspicion of ureteral or kidney injury.

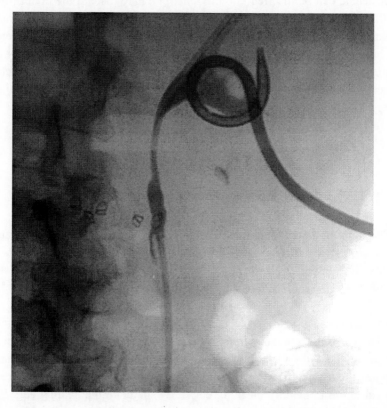

Figure 2. Retrograde pyelogram demonstrates mid- to proximal ureteral injury with extravasation of contrast. Patient was conservatively managed with ureteral stenting and nephrostomy tube drainage.

A one-shot IVP is performed by injecting 2mL/kg of intravenous contrast and taking an abdominal radiograph 10 minutes later. Contrast extravasation, ureteral dilation or absence, and delayed renal excretion are abnormal and can indicate injury. However, IVPs can have sensitivities as low as 61%, indicating that a negative IVP may warrant surgical exploration if the suspicion for ureteral injury remains high [1].

Retroperitoneal exploration is the most invasive but also the best method to diagnose ureteral injury with detection rates nearing 90% [18]. Direct visualization will reveal total or partial ureteral transection, ecchymosis, ischemia, and peristalsis. Peristalsis, however, does not preclude ureteral injury. If no injury is identified and suspicion remains high, intravenous indigo carmine or methylene blue may help identify the injury. Alternatively, a small caliber needle can be inserted into the renal pelvis to distend the ureter (much like filling a bladder via a urethral catheter) to identify fluid extravasation. A combination of retroperitoneal exploration with cystoscopy with ureteral cannulation and/or contrast injection is sometimes required to definitively rule out a ureteral injury. If the retrograde pyelogram is normal and the ureteral catheter passes easily into the renal pelvis, then a ureteral injury is highly unlikely.

Treatment

Overview

The most important factors in dictating surgical management of ureteral injuries are patient prognosis, associated injuries, and timing. In patients too unstable for definitive repair, ureteral ligation with nephrostomy tube placement is reasonable. Plans are made for ureteral reconstruction at a later date.

Very rarely, nephrectomy is an option, especially in cases of concomitant renal damage and irreparable ureter trauma. In stable patients, the location and extent of injury will dictate the type of surgical repair. There are four general principles: 1) preserve the ureteral blood supply during mobilization; 2) resect damaged tissue to healthy bleeding edges; 3) spatulate the healthy edges and anastomose with absorbable suture, preferably monofilament; 4) and place a ureteral stent.

Contusions

No urinary extravasation is seen in ureteral contusions, but ischemic damage may lead to ureteral stricture disease. If severe, resection of the damaged segment with primary anastomosis is ideal. Stenting may treat minor contusions, but it will only temporize more severe ones since stent removal will eventually lead to ureteral stricture and obstruction.

Partial Transections or Perforation

Partial ureteral injury via stab incisions do not have adjacent thermal injury and can therefore be repaired primarily. If possible, a horizontal closure of a longitudinal laceration can minimize the risk of stricture. Partial injuries from GSWs should not be repaired this way. Instead, the involved ureter segment with margins of 2cm should be resected to ensure removal of all thermally damaged tissue. The healthy ends are then reconnected with spatulation and anastomosis.

Upper Ureteral Injuries

Short proximal ureteral injuries can be repaired with ureteroureterostomy with internal stenting. Longer defects may require kidney mobilization, which involves dissecting completely around the kidney with inferior displacement and adherence to the psoas muscle. This will make up a distance of about 5cm.

To perform an ureteroureterostomy, the ureter is identified and mobilized. The injured segment is removed, ensuring healthy margins, with spatulation and placement of interrupted absorbable monofilament sutures (Figure 3). We prefer 5-0 polydioxanone on a small tapered needle and placement of a percutaneous drain near but not on the anastomosis. Drains can be removed when the output is low, typically on postoperative day 3 or 4. Complications of ureteroureterostomy include urine leakage, ileus, abscess, and fistula. Delayed complications include ureteral stricture. Leaks can be managed with percutaneous drainage and internal stenting. Strictures can be managed with endoscopic dilation and prolonged stenting, or open repair. The overall success rate is around 90%. Ureteropyelostomy is performed for traumas to the renal pelvis or proximal ureter, such as an avulsion injury (Figure 4). Ureterocalicostomy involves exposing a renal calyx—typically the lower pole calyx—and sewing the spatulated ureter to the calyx. This technique is indicated in traumas damaging the renal pelvis or UPJ beyond repair.

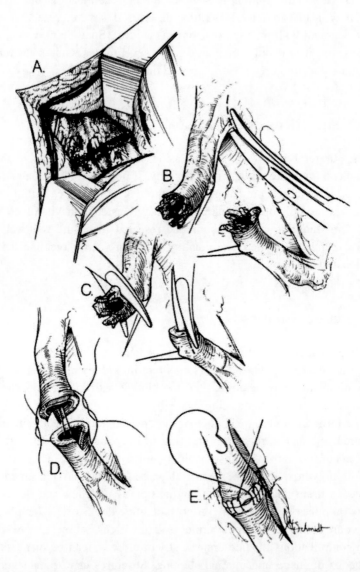

Figure 3. Damaged ureter segment is identified (A), exposed (B), resected and spatulated (C). The healthy ends are then brought together with interrupted or running absorbable suture (D + E).

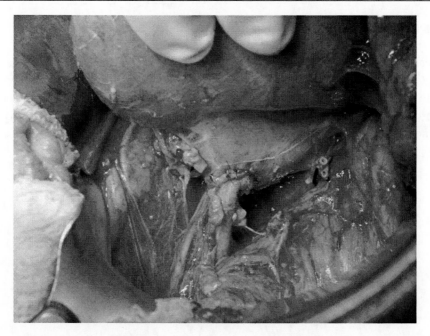

Figure 4. Primary anastomosis between the proximal ureter (spatulated) to the renal pelvis with interrupted monofilament absorbable suture.

Mid Ureteral Injuries

If short, mid ureteral injuries are also repaired with ureteroureterostomy as described before. If long or extensive, transureteroureterostomy can be considered. This procedure involves tunneling the injured ureter carefully thru an avascular portion of the sigmoid mesentery. The ureteral segment is then anastomosed to the healthy ureter in an end-to-side fashion. However, this procedure has been abandoned by most reconstructive urologists as there are other alternatives that avoid putting the remaining healthy collecting system at risk. Examples include a psoas hitch, Boari flap, and even small bowel interposition.

Lower Ureteral Injuries

Ureteroneocystostomy is the procedure of choice for distal injuries. It can bridge defects up to 5cm. Principles of repair include ureteral and bladder

mobilization to ensure a tension-free anastomosis. A small opening is made
thru the detrusor muscle and bladder mucosa that matches the size of a
spatulated ureter. We prefer a location superior and medial to the ipsilateral
ureteral orifice to minimize kinking. Absorbable sutures are then used to sew
the ureter to the bladder. Non-refluxing technique requires tunneling the ureter
thru the mucosa of the bladder with a backing of detrusor muscle (Figure 5).
The ratio of tunnel length to ureter diameter should be 3:1. This often has to be
performed intravesically thru an anterior cystotomy.

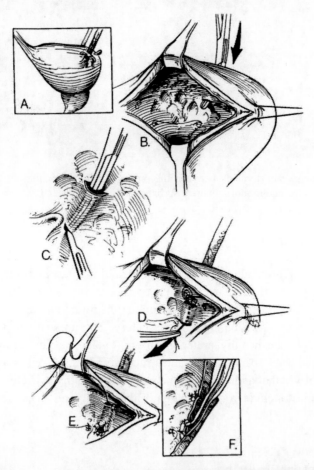

Figure 5. A. Location of bladder opening is superior and medial to the native ureter. B.
Cystotomy exposes the mucosa. C. Submucosal tunnel is developed. D. Suture is
secured to the distal ureter and brought thru the tunnel. E. The ureter is sewn to the
bladder in an interrupted fashion. F. Intramural view of ureteral reimplantation into the
bladder.

For longer distal ureteral injuries, a vesicopsoas hitch can be performed. The bladder is mobilized and pulled superiorly and laterally. Sometimes the contralateral superior vesical arteries and umbilicus are transected and ligated to improve bladder mobilization. The bladder is then fixed to the surface of the psoas muscle and tendon with thick absorbable suture, taking care not to injure the nearby genitofemoral and femoral nerves. Occasionally, a horizontal anterior cystotomy is made followed by vertical closure to improve superior dislocation of the bladder (Figure 6). The psoas bladder hitch can bridge a 6-8cm ureteral defect.

For very long segments of injured distal ureter, a Boari flap can be created. This technique involves making a broad based anterior bladder flap and tubularizing it with absorbable suture (Figure 7).

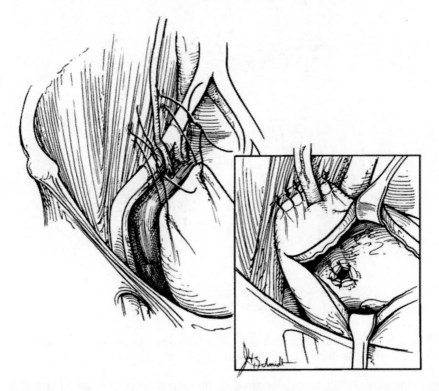

Figure 6. Vesicopsoas hitch. The bladder is secured to the psoas muscle with interrupted suture. An anterior cystotomy facilitates ureteral reimplantation and bladder mobilization.

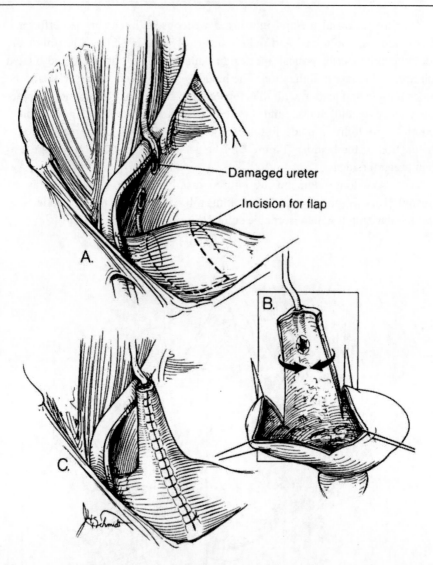

Damaged ureter

Incision for flap

A.

B.

C.

Figure 7. Boari flap. An anterior bladder flap is identified (A), mobilized (B), and then tubularized (C) to bridge the gap to the remaining ureteral segment.

The tubularized flap is then secured to the psoas tendon. A Boari flap can bridge a 12cm defect. Emphasis must be placed on not performing this procedure as it is rarely required, timely to perform (and therefore not appropriate in the acute trauma setting), and wrought with complications.

All of these techniques require bladder drainage with a urethral catheter and/or suprapubic tube, followed by a cystogram in 7-10 days to verify adequate bladder healing. Ureteral stents are left in place for 6 weeks prior to removal. Animal studies suggest that 6-8 weeks of ureteral stenting will allow mucosal (3weeks) and muscular (7 weeks) healing [19].

Complications include bladder ischemia, ureteral stricture, anastomotic stricture, urinary leakage, infection, and renal failure. Small capacity high pressure bladders from obstruction or neuropathic etiologies would make repair difficult; they also increase the risks of renal failure and pyelonephritis.

Extensive Ureteral Injuries

Pan-ureteral injuries are rarely seen in the trauma setting. Specific and extremely infrequent situations include ureteroscopic avulsion injuries, injection of sclerosing agent inadvertently into the ureter, radiation damage, and retroperitoneal fibrosis. Options for management include renal autotransplantation, ureteral substitution, or urinary diversion.

Autotransplantation involves removing the ipsilateral kidney, renal artery, renal vein, and renal pelvis and remaining healthy ureter down to the lower abdominal quadrant and anastomosing the renal vessels to the iliac vessels and the renal pelvis/ureter to the bladder.

Urologists are more familiar with small bowel surgery than kidney transplantation. For this reason and others (avoiding vascular anastomoses), we prefer ureteral substitution with ileal interposition over autotransplantation. Ileal ureter substitution involves isolating a segment of ileum much like in bowel harvest during ileal conduit creation. The main difference is the use of a longer segment (about 20cm).

The ileal segment is not tapered to minimize strictures. Left sided substitutions will need reflection of the descending colon and tunneling thru the sigmoid mesentery. Right sided repair requires reflection of the ascending colon. The distal end of the segment is anastomosed to the bladder in a simple refluxing anastomotic fashion with interrupted absorbable suture without internal stenting (Figure 8). Contraindications to the ileal ureter include serum creatinine greater than 2mg/dL, bladder outlet obstruction, neurogenic bladder, and liver disease. Complications include metabolic disturbances from absorption of urine, pyelonephritis, and mucous obstruction. Carefully choosing patients for this surgery will avoid ileal segment obstruction with resultant hyperchloremic hypokalemic metabolic acidosis. Detailed postoperative instructions can minimize mucous plugging.

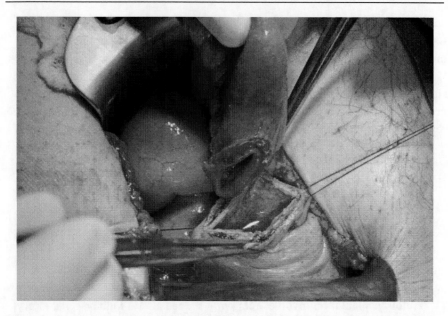

Figure 8. Segment of ileum is anastomosed to the bladder distally. No ileal tapering is performed to minimize risk of stricture.

Awareness of chronic bacteriuria and the need for adequate bladder emptying will reduce incidences of pyelonephritis. With an overall patency rate of over 90% [20], younger, healthier patients with severe ureteral disease should not be managed with chronic ureteral stents or nephrostomy tubes. They should be offered ileal ureter replacement.

Urinary diversion with ureteral stents or percutaneous nephrostomy is appropriate for patients with dire prognoses, who refuse surgery, or who are unfit for surgery.

Prevention of Iatrogenic Ureteral Injuries

Intraoperative ureteral stenting does not help decrease ureteral injury in gynecologic [21] or pelvic general surgery [22]. One general surgery study demonstrated that stents were considered "helpful" by the surgeon in 27% of pelvic cases [23]. Lighted fiberoptic stents help identify the ureter during laparoscopic surgery [24]. Despite stenting, injury still occurred in 1.6% of cases, and therefore stents are not generally recommended [25]. Stents do, however, increase intraoperative recognition of ureteral injury [26]. Having stents though, may actually increase the chance of ureteral injury [27]. Complications from intraoperative stents include hematuria and even renal failure in up to 5-6% of cases [24, 28]. Of note, a single study found ureteral catheters helpful preoperatively with low complication rates [29]. Maneuvers that help to avoid ureteral injury include open inspection and meticulous control of bleeding (to improve visualization) [30, 31].

Conclusion

Ureteral trauma is a rare event. Iatrogenic ureteral injury is less rare. Management varies greatly and depends on location and severity of disease, as well as concomitant injuries. Options include ureteral stent placement, percutaneous nephrostomy, ureteroneocystostomy, ureteroureterostomy, vesicopsoas hitch, Boari flap, and ileal ureter substitution. Intraoperative stenting for pelvic surgery does not decrease the risk of ureteral injury but it may improve its detection.

References

[1] Elliott SP; McAninch JW. Ureteral injuries from external violence: the 25-year experience at San Francisco General Hospital. *J. Urol*, 2003; 170: 1213-6.

[2] Best CD; Petrone P; Buscarini M; Demiray S; Kuncir E; Kimbrell B; Asensio JA. Traumatic ureteral inuries: a single institution experience validating the American Association for Surgery of Trauma-Organ Injury Scale grading scale. *J. Urol*, 2005; 173: 1202-5.

[3] Cinman NM, McAninch JW, Porten SP, Myers JB, Blaschko SD, Bagga HS, Breyer BN. Gunshot wounds to the lower urinary tract: a single-institution experience. *J. Trauma Acute Care Surg.* 2013;74:725-30.

[4] Mulligan JM, Cagiannos I, Collins JP, Millward SF. Ureteropelvic junction disruption secondary to blunt trauma: excretory phase imaging (delayed films) should help prevent a missed diagnosis. *J. Urol.* 1998; 159:67-70.

[5] Howerton RA, Norwood SN. Proximal ureteral avulsion from blunt abdominal trauma. *Miltary Med.* 1991; 156:311.

[6]   Hall SJ; Carpinito GA. Traumatic rupture of a renal pelvis obstructed at
       the ureteropelvic junction: case report. *J. Trauma*, 1994; 37: 850-2.

[7]   Lynch TH; Martinez-Pinero L; Plas E; Serafetinides E; Turkeri L;
       Santucci RA; Hohenfellner M. European Association of Urology. EAU
       guidelines on urological trauma. *Eur. Urol*, 2005; 47: 1-15.

[8]   Harkki-Siren P; Sjoberg J; Tiitinen A. Urinary tract injuries after
       hysterectomy. *Obstet. Gynecol*, 1998; 92: 113-8.

[9]   Ostrzenski A; Radolinski B; Ostrzenska KM. A review of laparoscopic
       ureteral injury in pelvic surgery. *Obstet. Gynecol. Surv*, 2003; 58: 794-9.

[10]   Parpala-Sparman T; Paananen I; Santala M; Ohtonen P; Hellstrom P.
       Increasing numbers of ureteric injuries after the introduction of
       laparoscopic surgery. *Scand. J. Urol. Nephrol*, 2008; 42: 422-7.

[11]   Lim MC; Lee BY; Lee DO; Joung JY; Kang S; Seo SS; Chung J; Park
       SY. Lower urinary tract injuries diagnosed after hysterectomy: seven
       year experience at a cancer hospital. *J. Obstet. Gynaecol. Res*, 2010;
       36:318-25.

[12]   Mathevet P; Valencia P; Cousin C; Mellier G; Dargent D. Operative
       injuries during vaginal hysterectomy. *Eur. J. Obstet. Gynecol. Reprod.
       Biol*, 2001; 97:71-5.

[13]   Coburn M. Ureteral injuries from surgical trauma. In: McAninch
       JW. *Traumatic and Reconstructive Urology*. Philadelphia, PA: WB
       Saunders Co; 1996:181-97.

[14]   Palaniappa NC, Telem DA, Ranasinghe NE, Divino CM. Incidence of
       iatrogenic ureteral injury after laparoscopic colectomy. *Arch. Surg.*
       2012;147:267-71.

[15]   Selzman AA; Spirnak JP. Iatrogenic ureteral injuries: a 20-yr experience
       in treating 165 injuries. *J. Urol*, 1996; 155:878-81.

[16]   Traxer O, Thomas A. Prospective evaluation and classification of
       ureteral wall injuries resulting from insertion of a ureteral access sheath
       during retrograde intrarenal surgery. *J. Urol.* 2013; 189:580-4.

[17]   Martov AG, Gurbanov ShSh, Tokareva EV, Shcherbinin SN, Kornienko
       SI. Comparison of the results of magnetic resonance urography and
       other examination methods in patients with iatrogenic injuries of the
       ureter and pelvis-ureteral segment. *Urologiia* 2009.;3:7-12.

[18]   Digiacomo JC, Frankel H, Rotondo MF, Schwab CW, Shaftan GW.
       Preoperative radiographic staging for ureteral injuries is not warranted in
       patients undergoing celiotomy for trauma. *Am. Surg.* Oct 2001;10:
       969-73.

[19] Andreoni CR, Lin HK, Olweny E, Landman J, Lee D, Bostwick D. Comprehensive evaluation of ureteral healing after electrosurgical endopyelotomy in a porcine model: original report and review of the literature. *J. Urol.* 2004;171:859-69.

[20] Bonfig R, Gerharz EW, Riedmiller H. Ileal ureteric replacement in complex reconstruction of the urinary tract. *BJU Int.* 2004; 93:575-80.

[21] Kuno K, Menzin A, Kauder HH, Sison C, Gal D. Prophylactic ureteral catheterization in gynecologic surgery. *Urology* 1988; 52: 1004-8.

[22] Bothwell WN, Bleicher RJ, Dent TL. Prophylactic ureteral catheterization in colon surgery. A five year review. *Dis. Colon Rectum* 1994; 37:330-4.

[23] Kyzer S, Gordon PH. The prophylactic use of ureteral catheters during colorectal operations. *Am. Surg.* 1994; 60:212-6.

[24] Chahin F, Dwivedi AJ, Paramesh A, Chau W, Agrawal S, Chahin C, Jumar A, Tootla A, Toola F, Silva YJ. The implications of lighted ureteral stenting in laparoscopic colectomy. *Jsls* 2002; 6:49-52.

[25] Symmonds RE. Ureteral injuries associated with gynecologic surgery: prevention and management. *Clin. Obstet. Gynecol.* 1976; 23:76-90.

[26] Leff EI, Groff W, Rubin RJ, Eisenstat TE, Salvati EP. Use of ureteral catheters in colonic and rectal surgery. *Dis. Colon. Rectum.* 1982; 25:457-60.

[27] Shingleton HM. Repairing injuries to the urinary tract: update on general surgery. *Contemp. Obstet. Gynecol.* 1984; 23:76-90.

[28] Sheikh FA, Khubchandani IT. Prophylactic ureteric catheters in colon surgery—how safe are they? Report of 3 cases. *Dis. Colon. Rectum.* 1990; 33:508-10.

[29] Quinlan DJ, Townsend DE, Johnson GH. Are ureteral catheters in gynecologic surgery beneficial or hazardous? *J. Am. Assoc. Gynecol. Laparosc.* 1995; 3-61-66.

[30] Cruikshank SH. Surgical method of identifying the ureters during total vaginal hysterectomy. *South Med. J.* 1985;78:1447-50.

[31] Liapis A, Bakas P, Giannopoulos V, Creatsas G. Ureteral injuries during gynecological surgery. *Int. Urogynecol. J. Pelvic. Floor Dysfunct.* 2001;12:391-3.

In: Ureters: Anatomy, Physiology and Disorders   ISBN: 978-1-62808-874-8
Editors: R. A. Santucci and M. Chen   © 2013 Nova Science Publishers, Inc.

Chapter 3

Endoscopic Management of Urolithiasis

Takashi Kawahara,[1,2,3,*] *Hiroki Ito,*[2,3]
Hiroshi Miyamoto,[1] *Hiroji Uemura,*[2]
Yoshinobu Kubota[2] *and Junichi Matsuzaki*[3]

[1]Department of Surgical Pathology and Laboratory Medicine,
University of Rochester Medical Center, Rochester, NY, US
[2]Department of Urology, Yokohama City University
Graduate School of Medicine, Yokohama, Kanagawa, Japan
[3]Department of Urology, Ohguchi Higashi General
Hospital, Yokohama, Kanagawa, Japan

Abstract

The development of rigid and flexible ureteroscopy (URS) has advanced the field of endoscopic ureteral surgery. Adjunct tools that facilitate endoscopic management include ureteral access sheaths (UAS), ureteral stents, basket devices for retrieving stone fragments, and fiber optic laser fibers.

* Corresponding author: Takashi Kawahara M.D. Department of Urology, Ohguchi Higashi General Hospital, 2-19-1, Irie, Kanagawa-ku, Yokohama, Kanagawa, Japan. E-mail: takashi_tk2001@yahoo.co.jp; Facsimile: +81-45-431-6920; Phone: +81-45-401-2411.

Ureteral stents are a fundamental part of many urological endoscopic procedures. They play a prominent role in management of obstructive ureteral stones, ureteral strictures, ureteropelvic junction obstruction, and retroperitoneal tumors or fibrosis. Stents also help dilate the ureter, thereby increasing the rates of successfully inserting an UAS. However, the long-term use of indwelling ureteral stents may also be associated with serious complications, such as encrustation, incrustation, and infection. Less serious adverse effects include bothersome urinary symptoms like urgency, frequency, lower abdominal cramping, and dysuria.

The use of UAS facilitates URS and retrieval of stone fragments, while also reducing intrarenal pressure, improving irrigation flow, and thereby decreasing the length of such operations. The problem with UAS is its potential to induce ureteral stricture as a result of ureteral mucosal ischemia.

This chapter describes our experience in endoscopic management of urolithiasis.

Ureteroscopy

In 1964, Marshall first reported the use of flexible ureteroscopy (URS). [1] Subsequently, in 1971, Takagi et al. reported the use of passively deflectable flexible URS. [2] In recent years, major advances have made observation of the ureter and renal pelvis easier, and it is now possible to perform a wide variety of intrarenal procedures using URS. [3] The ureteral access sheath (UAS) can facilitate ureteroscopic movement in and out of the ureter, improving the surgeon's ability to treat diseases such as ureteral and kidney stones. The UAS, by reducing intrarenal pressure and by improving irrigant flow, has no doubt contributed to the advancement of ureteroscopy. [4-6]

Ureteroscopic Lithotripsy

El-Anany et al. showed that endoscopic access and complete stone fragmentation can be achieved in 77% of patients using a Holmium Yattrium Aluminum Garnet (Ho: YAG) laser. [7] Prior EAU and AUA Nephrolithiasis Guidelines recommend rigid URS as the first-line treatment for small, less than 10mm, ureteral stones, but not renal stones. [4, 8-11] However, with the development of smaller caliber semirigid and flexible ureteroscopes, URS has become a safer and more established modality for treating all types of urinary stones.

Based on evidence of the efficacy of the presented technique, we have performed ureteroscopic lithotripsy even when the diameter of the stone is greater than 15 mm. [12]

To predict stone-free rates, we evaluated stone characteristics by measuring size and density (Hounsfield units) on CT. [8, 13] Our previous study showed that using one cutoff point for the stone volume and surface area is most effective for predicting the outcome of URS. These cutoff values are: 1) traced surface area (tSA) <110.0 mm^2; 2) calculated surface area (cSA) <125.0 mm^2; and 3) stone volume < 840 mm^3. These cutoff points are significant predictors of stone-free rates. [8, 13]

The detailed technique of ureteroscopic lithotripsy is described in our previous reports. [4, 8, 9, 12]

Briefly, under general anesthesia, the patient is placed in the lithotomy position. A 6-Fr rigid URS (Uretero-Renoscope®, Karl Storz, Germany) is inserted into the ureter toward the renal pelvis under guidewire assistance; this allows us to evaluate the entire ureter.

Leaving the guidewire in place, we withdraw the rigid ureteroscope and insert a UAS into the ureter under fluoroscopic guidance, and then perform flexible URS to evaluate the renal pelvis and calyces. Intracorporeal lithotripsy is carried out with a Ho:YAG laser via 550- to 200-micrometer laser fibers passed through a rigid or flexible URS scope. The stone fragments were retrieved using nitinol baskets.

The flexible URS scopes used included the Flex X2 (Karl Stortz, Germany) and P5 (Olympus, Japan). The UAS used included the FLEXOR (Cook Urological, US) with an inner and outer diameter of 14/16-Fr and 12/14-Fr, respectively, and the Navigator (Boston Scientific, US) with an inner and outer diameter of 13/15-Fr and 11/13-Fr, respectively. The length of the UAS was 35 cm for the FLEXOR and 46 cm for the Navigator. The laser fibers included SlimLine (LUMENIS surgical, US) with a diameter of 200, 365 or 550 micrometers. The laser generators included 30W or 100W Ho:YAG lasers (VersaPulse 30W and VersaPulse PowerSuite 100W, LUMENIS surgical, US). The nitinol stone retrieval baskets included the 1.5-Fr N-circle (Cook Urological, US) and the 1.9-Fr ZeroTip (BostonScientific, US). Ureteral stents or ureteral catheters were placed at the conclusion of all ureteroscopic procedures.

In addition, based on the preliminary study of the laser power settings in patients with bladder stones, we are now investigating the correlation between the laser power settings using the Ho: YAG laser and the stone-free rates associated with these settings. [14]

Ureteral Access Sheath (UAS)

The use of a UAS is necessary to perform endoscopic procedures in the upper ureter and renal collecting system. The sheath reduces intrarenal pressure and improves stone-free rates. It also decreases incidence of postoperative urinary tract infections [15, 16]. Previous studies have shown that preoperative stenting facilitates UAS insertion and achieves higher stone-free rates compared with that observed in patients who are not stented preoperatively [12]. In addition, some patients who are not able to undergo insertion of UAS into the ureter in the initial procedure are stented and successfully undergo UAS insertion during the followup procedure. For these reasons, ureteral stenting is thought to dilate the ureter.

To confirm the effectiveness of preoperative stenting, we conducted a study comparing intentional preoperative stenting and non-preoperative stenting among patients undergoing ureteroscopic lithotripsy for large renal stones. In this study, we excluded patients with hydronephrosis and positive urine cultures for the purpose of preventing patient selection bias. Consequently, the intentional preoperative stenting group exhibited a higher rate of success of large-caliber UAS insertion. We concluded that preoperative stenting dilates the ureter and facilitates subsequent UAS insertion, therefore resulting in a higher stone-free rate. [12]

Ureteroscopy-Assisted Retrograde Nephrostomy (UARN)

In the classical procedure of percutaneous nephrolithotomy (PCNL), ureteroscopic procedures are not performed except for the insertion of an occlusion balloon catheter to dilate the renal collecting system and the retrieval of kidney stones that migrated down the ureter during PCNL. Due to recent developments in ureteroscopic management, URS and ureteroscopic lithotripsy is sometimes used concomitantly with PCNL to optimally treat large kidney stones. Recent reports have shown that the combination of URS and PCNL achieves higher stone-free and effective rates than PCNL alone because URS can be used to detect and remove stones where a nephroscope cannot reach [17].

We previously reported the use of ureteroscopy-assisted retrograde nephrostomy (UARN) during PCNL. [18, 19]

Briefly, under general and epidural anesthesia, the patient was placed in a modified-Valdivia position (Galdakao-modified Valdivia position). [20] After inserting a ureteral access sheath, URS was performed to observe the renal collecting system and target stones. We confirmed the location of the target stones and determined the target calyx for puncture. A Lawson retrograde nephrostomy puncture wire (Cook Urological, US) was set via URS and directed towards the target calyx, which was subsequently punctured. Using UARN, the surgeon was able to achieve access by reaching the target puncture spot and then insert a nephron-access sheath (NAS) under visualization.

The use of URS during PCNL contributes to a higher stone-free rate, lower surgical times, and fewer complications. [21] Therefore, UARN is helpful for all kidney stone procedures; it is especially helpful for difficult cases like in patients who are obese, who have had prior renal surgery, or who have anatomic anomalies.

Obese Patients

Flexible ureteroscopic lithotripsy for obese patients has been reported to result in stone-free rates of approximately 70–100%. [22] However, due to the length of time required to create stone fragments and remove large stones, it has been suggested that patients with a greater stone burden would be better treated with PCNL. Indeed, PCNL is preferable in obese patients with large renal calculi (>2 cm). [23] As increased surgical morbidity and mortality is associated with obesity in general, PCNL is performed in the supine position for morbidly obese patients in order to minimize risks. [23] These problems result from the difficulty of making fine adjustments under fluoroscopic guidance in obese patients whose skin-to-stone distance is quite long. We showed that nephrostomy can be easily achieved in an ideal position, without the need for a position change from the lithotomy position to the prone position and vice versa using UARN. [24] We previously reported a case of renal calculi successfully treated with UARN during PCNL in an obese patient. [23]

Patients with an Ileal Conduit

The implementation of a diversion that requires the use of an appliance, such as an ileal conduit or cutaneous ureterostomy, is primarily considered for patients undergoing radical cystectomy who are not candidates for continent diversion procedures. [25] However, a significant number of patients present with complications associated with ileal conduit diversion. In addition, ureteral calculi have been reported to develop at later stages in 10.7% of patients, and ureteroileal obstruction has been reported to occur in 4% to 7.9% of patients. [26] As described by JD Schmidt et al., ureteral calculi develop in 10.7% of patients in the later postoperative period. [27] Turk et al. reported that urinary stone formation is one of the more common adverse events and can develop in the upper urinary tract or within the diversion itself in up to 11% of patients within three years after surgery. [28] An antegrade or retrograde approach can be used to achieve access to the ureter in individuals with ileal conduit urinary diversion. [29] PCNL is often considered the treatment of first choice to achieve a stone-free status in patients with urinary diversions and large or complex upper tract calculi. However, in patients with non-dilated renal collecting systems, puncturing and inserting the guidewire into the ureter is sometimes challenging. We treated three patients with renal stones and ileal conduits (created in Bricker fashion) in whom we performed PCNL using UARN. In these patients, we also successfully inserted UAS without any difficulty. [30] That being said, it is notoriously difficult to access the ureters retrograde in patients with ureteroileal anastomoses, and antegrade access is preferable.

Patients Who Have Undergone Anatrophic Nephrolithotripsy (ANL)

Open surgical anatrophic nephrolithotomy (ANL) was the standard treatment for large renal stones prior to the development of endoscopic procedures. The surgical management of urinary calculi disease has evolved from an open surgical approach to various minimally invasive options, including URS, SWL and PCNL. [31, 32] The treatment of patients with staghorn calculi remains among the most complex and challenging problems in urology. [33] ANL with formal calyorrhaphy and/or calycoplasty was first described by Smith and Boyce in 1968. [34]

Matlaga and Assimos reported a stone-free rate of 100% using open stone surgery for staghorn renal stones. [35] Kaouk et al. were the first to report experience with laparoscopic ANL in a porcine model. [36] ANL is recognized to be more reliable than SWL or PCNL in terms of stone removal when treating large staghorn calculi, with stone-free rates of 80-100%. [37, 38]

Performing repeated ANL for recurrent renal stones is difficult due to the invasiveness of ANL and postoperative adhesions. Goodwin et al. first reported percutaneous renal access in 1955. [39] The renal position was repositioned dorsally due to intraoperative separation and postoperative adhesions associated with ANL. As a result, obtaining access from the middle calyx on the dorsal side was too dorsal. The most critical issue in PCNL placement is selecting the proper puncture site in order to minimize the risk of hemorrhage, which is the most common major complication. Ultrasound (US)- or fluoroscopic-guided puncture of the collecting system with subsequent placement of the drainage tube is the standard modality for PCNL; however, performing US-guided nephrostomy is difficult in patients with anatomical anomalies of the abdomen or kidneys. Major advances with URS have made it possible to perform a wide variety of intrarenal procedures. [40] Therefore, it is easier to approach the desired renal calyx using a flexible URS scope than was possible using previous sonographic or fluoroscopic approaches. [41, 42] A potential disadvantage of this procedure is the danger of exiting the kidney ventrally and therefore increasing risk of injuring the intestines. [43] UARN is also a safe and effective approach for patients presenting with calculi after having previously undergone ANL. [44]

Patients with Incomplete Double Ureters

The incidence of a double renal pelvis and ureter ranges from 0.5% to 3.0% in humans. [45, 46] Anomalous duplication of the ureter and pelvis is classified as complete or incomplete. [45, 46] Incomplete duplication is three times more common than complete duplication. In incomplete duplication, the pelvis and two ureters join and enter the bladder via one common orifice. Such duplication may be unilateral or bilateral. Patients with duplication of the ureter have an increased risk of stone formation [47]. In our institute, we experienced two patients with incomplete double ureters who successfully underwent PCNL using UARN. UARN may represent a new option for performing PCNL in subjects with ureteral duplication. [48]

Patients with a Horseshoe Kidney

Horseshoe kidneys are the most common renal fusion anomalies, with a prevalence of 0.25% in the general population. [49]

Most horseshoe kidneys are fused by the formation of an isthmus between the lower poles of the left and right kidneys during development. [50] SWL, URS, PCNL and open surgery are used to treat renal stones in patients with horseshoe kidneys. [49-52] Some patients with horseshoe kidneys have been successfully treated with ureteroscopy, although due to the altered anatomical relationships observed in patients with this disorder, the use of ureteroscopic approaches can be quite challenging and is not universally recommended. [52, 53] In several small case series, PCNL was shown to be highly successful, with an overall stone-free rate of 89%. [54] PCNL is also suitable for treating renal calculi in the lower calyx in patients with a horseshoe kidney. However, performing nephrostomy on the target calyx is difficult without dilating the renal collecting system even if an occlusion balloon catheter is used to create hydronephrosis. Nevertheless, the usefulness of PCNL for renal calculi in patients with horseshoe kidneys has been reported. [49, 54, 55, 56, 57]

Although the use of ureteroscopic lithotripsy for renal calculi in patients with horseshoe kidneys has been reported, accessing the lower pole with an ureteroscope is sometimes difficult due to higher insertion of the ureter into the renal collecting system. [49, 53]

To reach the lower calyx, nephrostomy is usually created in the upper calyx. Among patients with a horseshoe kidney, Raj et al. reported that 15 of 24 patients (64%) required nephrostomy in the upper calyx, and Al-Otabi et al. reported that nine of 12 patients (75%) required this specific access point. [49, 54] The use of an upper pole nephrostomy tract allows for enhanced intrarenal access to the upper pole calyx, renal pelvis, lower pole calyx, ureteropelvic junction and proximal ureter. [49] The disadvantage of nephrostomy in the upper calyx is that it sometimes involves longer distances from the skin to the lower calyx, meaning that the nephroscope cannot reach the target stone. [49, 51] Moreover, Raj et al. reported a 6% rate of pneumothorax complications in patients undergoing nephrostomy in the upper calyx. [49] Clearly, an accurate puncture location in the upper calyx is required. We performed preoperative CT in all cases and performed US before puncture to avoid injuring the surrounding organs. Our procedure may make percutaneous nephrostomy possible and easy to perform. A previous report described PCNL as a safe and established procedure, although severe complications requiring blood transfusions and chest tubes can sometimes occur. [58] At our institute, URS was successful in treating a number of cases of renal calculi in the lower calyx in patients with horseshoe kidneys. In these cases, we usually positioned the patient in the Galdakao-modified Valdivia position and performed URS initially to confirm whether the URS could reach the target stone.

When it did not reach the target stone, percutaneous puncture under sonographic or fluoroscopic guidance was performed. Meanwhile, in all cases, UARN afforded accurate puncture based on ureteroscopic findings. In UARN, after the needle exited through the skin, no further steps were required in preparation for dilation. [41, 43]

UARN is a promising procedure that allows for accurate puncture of the desired calyx and is expected to contribute to optimal nephrostomy placement in the upper calyx for PCNL in patients with horseshoe kidneys. [59] We successfully performed PCNL using UARN in three patients whose renal stones were in the lower pole of their horseshoe kidney. [59]

Patients with a Complete Staghorn Stone

Partial staghorn calculi are branched, and sometimes infected stones that occupy a large portion of the renal collecting system; complete staghorn calculi occupy the entire collecting system.

Complete staghorn calculi are typically treated with PCNL; however, performing dilating nephrostomy and inserting an Nephro Access SheathNAS can be difficult when there is no hydronephrosis, even when using an occlusion balloon catheter and ureteral catheter to create hydronephrosis. [60, 61] UARN can be effective in obtaining percutaneous renal collecting system access in cases of complete staghorn calculi. [62]

UARN without UAS

During UARN, we generally performed URS with a UAS; however, in two cases, we performed URS without UAS. UAS decreases intrarenal pressure and allows the URS to be controlled more easily.

However, using UAS carries a potential risk of ureteral mucosa ischemia and resultant ureteral stricture.

We attempted to perform UARN without UAS in four cases; however, two cases were aborted due to poor visualization and inability to approach the desired calix. Therefore, further studies of performing UARN without UAS are needed.

Ureteral Stents and Complications

Ureteral Stents

The first indwelling ureteral splint was described by Zimskind et al. in 1967. [63] Ureteral stents are now a fundamental part of many urological procedures performed for obstructing ureteral calculi, ureteral stricture, ureteropelvic junction obstruction and retroperitoneal tumors or fibrosis that develop after open or endoscopic ureteral surgery. [62, 64-66] The use of stents can result in unpleasant side effects, such as urinary frequency, urgency, incontinence, hematuria, bladder pain and flank pain, which have a negative impact on the patient's quality of life. [66-70]

Ureteral Stent Encrustation

Ureteral stents can be associated with serious complications, including migration, fragmentation and stone formation, especially when the stents are inadvertently forgotten. [64, 71, 72, 73] Ureteral stent encrustation, in particular, is the most devastating complication. A report by el-Faqih et al. indicated that the stent encrustation rate increases with time from 9.2% for less than six weeks to 47.5% at six to 12 weeks to 76.3% at more than 12 weeks. [74] Our previous reports also support this data. [75]

Bultitude et al. reported that 42.8% of stents become difficult to remove cystoscopically within four months, with 14.3% becoming difficult to remove at two months. [71, 76] Okuda et al. reported the cases of 15 irremovable ureteral stents in Japanese patients. The mean indwelling time of these stents was 20 months. [77] In our experience, patients with heavily encrusted ureteral stents must undergo ureteroscopic procedures to remove the encrusted ureteral stent. [78] Rarely, forgotten ureteral stents are sometimes smoothly removed without the need for any invasive procedures. [79]

We investigated a total of 330 ureteral stents in 181 patients for encrustation, incrustation, coloring and resistance to removal. The stent encrustation rate was 26.8% at less than six weeks, 56.9% at six to 12 weeks and 75.9% at more than 12 weeks in the present study. Among all stents, 46

(13.9%) were resistant to removal, and three of these could not be removed endoscopically. [80]

The mechanisms underlying stent coloration have not yet been proven, either in the present study or in previous studies.

However, most urologists have experienced coloration of ureteral stents and sometimes note that colored ureteral stents tend to be encrusted. [80]

Ureteral Stents and Ureteral Stent-Related Symptoms

Ureteral Stent-Related Symptoms

Ureteral stents carry a potential risk of ureteral stent-related symptoms, such as urinary frequency, urgency, incontinence, hematuria, bladder pain and flank pain, which have a negative impact on the patient's quality of life. [81-83]

Predicting the Ureteral Length

Choosing the optimal length of a ureteral stent is important for decreasing the incidence of stent migration and other complications, including ureteral stent-related symptoms. [84-87] Accurately predicting the ureteral length is required to determine the ideal ureteral stent length. [84, 87] In previous studies, the actual ureteral length was determined using direct measurement with a ureteral catheter and guidewire. [88, 89] Choosing a ureteral stent using direct measurement is ideal; however, direct measurement is associated with extra radiation exposure and extra procedures for both the patient and operator. Therefore, estimating the ureteral length is required. To estimate the patient's ureteral length, the correlation with the patient's height is generally used. However, the reliability of this method as an estimate of the ureteral length has not been confirmed. [89] We investigated the reliability of accurately approximating the ureteral length using multiple modalities in the same patient group. In addition, we developed a formula to estimate the ureteral length.

We measured a total of 169 ureteral stent lengths in 151 patients, which is the largest number ever published.

In this study, we confirmed that predicting the ureteral length using CT is better than using body height or intravenous pyelography. The detailed methods are described in our previous study. [90] Briefly, we used the Axial CT distance (ACTD). The ACTD was defined as the number of slices according to the interval of each slice on axial CT.

The upper slice was defined as the level of the renal vein and the lower slice was defined as the level of the UVJ. The estimated ureteral length was calculated from each variable as follows: estimated ureteral length (cm): 0.044 x ACTD (mm) + 13.25. Using this method, choosing an appropriate length of ureteral stent without invasive techniques is possible.

Correlation between the Ureteral Length and Stent Position

Choosing the optimal length of a ureteral stent is important for decreasing the incidence of stent migration and other complications. [84-87] Accurately predicting the ureteral length is required to determine the ideal stent length. [84, 87] Choosing a ureteral stent based on direct measurement is ideal; however, the relationship between the ureteral length and the ureteral stent length is unclear. We researched the relationship between the actual ureteral length and the ureteral stent position. [70]

We investigated the ureteral stent position in 226 cases and assessed the correlation between the ureteral stent position and the ureteral length measured using a loop type ureteral stent. The appropriate length of ureteral stent was the same or 1 cm less than the measured ureteral length. On the other hand, ureteral stents that are more than 2 cm smaller than the measured ureteral length are associated with an increased incidence of migration. Choosing an appropriate length of ureteral stent is difficult when the proximal end of the stent is in the upper calyx. There is an 11.0% risk that a ureteral stent the length of the ureteral length will be too long if the proximal end of the stent is located in the renal pelvis. A ureteral stent 1 cm shorter than the ureteral length has a 2.6% risk of migration and an 8.6% risk of being too long. [70]

Types of Ureteral Stents

Urinary stents contain various materials and are available in different sizes, coatings and shapes to avoid unpleasant urinary symptoms and discomfort. [91-93] It is necessary to minimize the amount of material in the bladder in order to decrease the incidence of stent-related symptoms. [91] Therefore, the Tail Stent® (Boston Scientific, US) was developed with a 7-Fr proximal pigtail at the proximal end and a 7-Fr shaft that tapers to a lumenless straight 3-Fr tail at the distal end. [94] Dunn et al. showed that the 7-Fr tail loop stent produces significantly less irritating symptoms than the standard 7-Fr double-pigtail stent. Lingeman et al. evaluated stent-related symptoms using a self-administered questionnaire for various types of ureteral stents. The loop-type ureteral stent was associated with a lower stent-related symptom score than the standard double stent; however, the difference was not significant. [91]

We investigated the incidence of stent-related symptoms after changing from a double-pigtail stent to a loop-type ureteral stent in the same patient group. [70] In this study, we compared the incidence of ureteral stent-related symptoms in 25 patients who changed from a double-pigtail ureteral stent to a loop-type ureteral stent. The incidences of almost all of the stent-related symptoms, other than nocturia, were significantly lower when the patients had loop-type ureteral stents than when the patients had double-pigtail stents. [70]

Ureteral Stent Removal and Exchange Using the Crochet Hook Technique

Temporary ureteral stenting is the standard procedure performed at the conclusion of most ureteroscopic procedures. For chronic ureteral diseases like stricture and retroperitoneal fibrosis, patients who are unfit for surgery require ureteral stents that are removed and/or exchanged every several months. However, ureteral stent removal or exchange requires the use of cystoscopy. Cystoscopy is a useful tool for grasping the distal end of the ureteral stent under visualization. Due to the invasiveness of cystoscopy, some patients do not come to the hospital for ureteral stent removal, and forgotten ureteral stents are sometimes seen in clinical practice. [78, 79] Therefore, in our institute, the crochet hook technique is used for female patients for the purpose of decreasing the incidence of ureteral stent-related symptoms.

A crochet hook is used in knitting to create fabric and knit patterns from yarn, including sweaters. Crochet hooks come in many sizes and materials, with a variety of hook sizes. Crochet hooks made of metal were selected and sterilized via autoclaving. Two percent lidocaine gel was spread on the hook, which was then inserted into the urethra. We primarily used a No. 4.5 crochet hook made of metal, which is the same diameter as a 7.5-Fr ureteral catheter.

Ureteral stent exchange is usually performed with both fluoroscopic and cystoscopic guidance.

Ureteral stent exchange using the crochet hook technique under fluoroscopic guidance without cystoscopy was first presented by Sakamoto, and we confirmed the effectiveness of this procedure. [95]

The details of the crochet hook exchange technique were described in our previous report. [95] Briefly, the crochet hook was advanced toward the ureteral orifice and carefully passed from the ureteral orifice to the urethra and passed gently over the bladder mucosa under fluoroscopic guidance. After the stent was passed from the external urethral orifice, a 0.035-inch guidewire was inserted into the ureteral stent. The old stent was removed and the new stent was inserted under fluoroscopic guidance. Performing ureteral stent exchange using a crochet hook under fluoroscopic guidance is easy, safe, and cost-effective. [96]

Ureteral stent removal using the crochet hook technique does not require cystoscopy or fluoroscopy. The details of the crochet hook technique were described in our previous report. [96] Briefly, lidocaine gel (2%) was spread on the hook, and the crochet hook was inserted into the urethra. The crochet hook was advanced toward the ureteral orifice and carefully passed from the ureteral orifice to the urethra and passed softly over the bladder mucosa. The surgeon repeated the same procedure several times until the distal end of the stent passed from the external urethral orifice. Performing ureteral stent removal using a crochet hook is easy and safe. This procedure does not require fluoroscopy or cystoscopy. This technique is easily acquired and is suitable for use on an outpatient basis. The results of our study showed that removal of ureteral stents using the crochet hook technique is usually well tolerated with minimal complications. [96]

Postoperative Ureteral Stricture

Despite the effectiveness of UAS for ureteroscopic lithotripsy, there is a potential risk of ureteral stricture. However, the detailed mechanisms remain unclear. Ureteral stricture is thought to result from ischemia of the ureteral mucosa caused by UAS. In a previous report, ischemia and pathological changes were found to be correlated with the duration of UAS in a pig model. To address these problems, we investigated the correlation between postoperative hydronephrosis and the duration of indwelling UAS. Our results showed that a longer dwell time is associated with a tendency toward the development of hydronephrosis within three days after surgery. However, despite the longer useof UAS, no patients developed ureteral stricture. Due to the low incidence of postoperative ureteral stricture, UAS is safe and effective. [97] Further studies are needed in the future to elaborate on the unconfirmed observation that prolonged UAS usage can lead to ureteral strictures.

Conclusion

Due to technologic advancements, ureteroscopic and nephroscopic management of urolithiasis has become safe and effective. As a result, stone disease of the urinary tract has evolved from an open surgical problem to a minimally invasive endoscopic one.

References

[1] Marshall, V. F. (1964) Fiber Optics in Urology. *J. Urol.* 91: 110-114.

[2] Takagi, T., Go, T., Takayasu, H., Aso, Y. (1971) Fiberoptic pyeloureteroscope. *Surgery* 70: 661-663 passim.

[3] Dasgupta, P., Cynk, M. S., Bultitude, M. F., Tiptaft, R. C., Glass, J. M. (2004) Flexible ureterorenoscopy: prospective analysis of the Guy's experience. *Ann. R Coll. Surg. Engl.* 86: 367-370.

[4] Ito, H., Kawahara, T., Terao, H., Ogawa, T., Yao, M., et al. (2013) Evaluation of preoperative measurement of stone surface area as a predictor of stone-free status after combined ureteroscopy with holmium laser lithotripsy: A single-center experience. *J. Endourol.*

[5] Monga, M., Bodie, J., Ercole, B. (2004) Is there a role for small-diameter ureteral access sheaths? Impact on irrigant flow and intrapelvic pressures. *Urology* 64: 439-441; discussion 441-432.

[6] Boddy, S. A., Nimmon, C. C., Jones, S., Ramsay, J. W., Britton, K. E., et al. (1988) Acute ureteric dilatation for ureteroscopy. An experimental study. *Br. J. Urol.* 61: 27-31.

[7] El-Anany, F. G., Hammouda, H. M., Maghraby, H. A., Elakkad, M. A. (2001) Retrograde ureteropyeloscopic holmium laser lithotripsy for large renal calculi. *BJU international* 88: 850-853.

[8] Ito, H., Kawahara, T., Terao, H., Ogawa, T., Yao, M., et al. (2012) Predictive value of attenuation coefficients measured as Hounsfield units

on noncontrast computed tomography during flexible ureteroscopy with holmium laser lithotripsy: a single-center experience. *J. Endourol.* 26: 1125-1130.

[9]   Ito, H., Kawahara, T., Terao, H., Ogawa, T., Yao, M., et al. (2012) The most reliable preoperative assessment of renal stone burden as a predictor of stone-free status after flexible ureteroscopy with holmium laser lithotripsy: a single-center experience. *Urology* 80: 524-528.

[10] Preminger, G. M., Tiselius, H. G., Assimos, D. G., Alken, P., Buck, C., et al. (2007) 2007 guideline for the management of ureteral calculi. *J. Urol.* 178: 2418-2434.

[11] Tiselius, H. G., Ackermann, D., Alken, P., Buck, C., Conort, P., et al. (2001) Guidelines on urolithiasis. *Eur. Urol.* 40: 362-371.

[12] Kawahara, T., Ito, H., Terao, H., Ishigaki, H., Ogawa, T., et al. (2012) Preoperative stenting for ureteroscopic lithotripsy for a large renal stone. *Int. J. Urol.* 19: 881-885.

[13] Kawahara, T., Ito, H., Terao, H., Ogawa, T., Uemura, H., et al. (2012) Stone area and volume are correlated with operative time for cystolithotripsy for bladder calculi using a holmium: yttrium garnet laser. *Scand. J. Urol. Nephrol.* 46: 298-303.

[14] Takashi Kawahara, H. I., Hideyuki Terao, Yoshitake Kato, Katsuyuki Tanaka, Takehiko Ogawa, Hiroji Uemura, Yoshinobu Kubota, Junichi Matsuzaki (2013) Correlation between the operation time using two different power settings of a Ho: YAG laser. *BMC Reserch Notes In press.*

[15] Monga, M. B. J., Ercole, B. (2004) Is there a role for small-diameter ureteral access sheath? Impact on irrigant flow and intrapelvic pressure. *Urology* 64: 439-441.

[16] Auge, B. K. P. P., Lallas, C. D., Raj, G. V., Santa-Cruz, R. W., Preminger, G. M. (2004) Ureteral access sheath provides protection against elevated renal pressures during routine flexible ureteroscopic stone manipulation. *J. Endourol.* 18: 33-36.

[17] Whyberg, J. B. B. J., Vicene, J. Z., Hannosh, V., Salmon, S. A. (2012) Flexible ureteroscopy-directed retrograde nephrostomy for percutaneous nephrolithotomy* description of a technique. *J. Endourol.* 26: 1268-1274.

[18] Kawahara, T., Ito, H., Terao, H., Yoshida, M., Ogawa, T., et al. (2012) Ureteroscopy assisted retrograde nephrostomy: a new technique for percutaneous nephrolithotomy (PCNL). *BJU Int.* 110: 588-590.

[19] Takashi Kawahara, H. I., Hideyuki Terao, Takehiko Ogawa, Hiroji Uemura, Yoshinobu Kubota, Junichi Matsuzaki (2012) Ureteroscopy-Assisted Retrograde Nephrostomy. *Journal of Endourology* Part B, Videourology 26: doi: 10.1089/vid.2011.0082.

[20] Valdivia Uria, J. G., Valle Gerhold, J., Lopez Lopez, J. A., Villarroya Rodriguez, S., Ambroj Navarro, C., et al. (1998) Technique and complications of percutaneous nephroscopy: experience with 557 patients in the supine position. *J. Urol.* 160: 1975-1978.

[21] Kawahara, T., Ito, H., Terao, H., Kato, Y., Uemura, H., et al. (2012) Effectiveness of ureteroscopy-assisted retrograde nephrostomy (UARN) for percutaneous nephrolithotomy (PCNL). *PLoS One* 7: e52149.

[22] Andreoni, C., Afane, J., Olweny, E., Clayman, R. V. (2001) Flexible ureteroscopic lithotripsy: first-line therapy for proximal ureteral and renal calculi in the morbidly obese and superobese patient. *J. Endourol.* 15: 493-498.

[23] Kang, D. E., Maloney, M. M., Haleblian, G. E., Springhart, W. P., Honeycutt, E. F., et al. (2007) Effect of medical management on recurrent stone formation following percutaneous nephrolithotomy. *J. Urol.* 177: 1785-1788; discussion 1788-1789.

[24] Kawahara, T., Matsuzaki, J., Kubota, Y. (2012) Ureteroscopy-assisted retrograde nephrostomy for an obese patient. *Indian J. Urol.* 28: 439-441.

[25] Rodriguez, A. R., Lockhart, A., King, J., Wiegand, L., Carrion, R., et al. (2011) Cutaneous ureterostomy technique for adults and effects of ureteral stenting: an alternative to the ileal conduit. *J. Urol.* 186: 1939-1943.

[26] Vandenbroucke, F., Van Poppel, H., Vandeursen, H., Oyen, R., Baert, L. (1993) Surgical versus endoscopic treatment of non-malignant uretero-ileal anastomotic strictures. *Br. J. Urol.* 71: 408-412.

[27] Schmidt, J. D., Hawtrey, C. E., Flocks, R. H., Culp, D. A. (1973) Complications, results and problems of ileal conduit diversions. *J. Urol.* 109: 210-216.

[28] Turk, T. M., Koleski, F. C., Albala, D. M. (1999) Incidence of urolithiasis in cystectomy patients after intestinal conduit or continent urinary diversion. *World J. Urol.* 17: 305-307.

[29] Drake, M. J., Cowan, N. C. (2002) Fluoroscopy guided retrograde ureteral stent insertion in patients with a ureteroileal urinary conduit: method and results. *J. Urol.* 167: 2049-2051.

[30] Kawahara, T., Ito, H., Terao, H., Ogawa, T., Uemura, H., et al. (2012) Ureteroscopy-assisted retrograde nephrostomy for percutaneous nephrolithotomy after urinary diversion. *Case Rep. Nephrol. Urol.* 2: 113-117.

[31] Zhou, L., Xuan, Q., Wu, B., Xiao, J., Dong, X., et al. (2011) Retroperitoneal laparoscopic anatrophic nephrolithotomy for large staghorn calculi. *Int. J. Urol.* 18: 126-129.

[32] Segura, J. W., Preminger, G. M., Assimos, D. G., Dretler, S. P., Kahn, R. I., et al. (1994) Nephrolithiasis Clinical Guidelines Panel summary report on the management of staghorn calculi. The American Urological Association Nephrolithiasis Clinical Guidelines Panel. *J. Urol.* 151: 1648-1651.

[33] Melissourgos, N. D., Davilas, E. N., Fragoulis, A., Kiminas, E., Farmakis, A. (2002) Modified anatrophic nephrolithotomy for complete staghorn calculus disease -- does it still have a place? *Scand. J. Urol. Nephrol.* 36: 426-430.

[34] Smith, M. J., Boyce, W. H. (1968) Anatrophic nephrotomy and plastic calyrhaphy. *J. Urol.* 99: 521-527.

[35] Matlaga, B. R., Assimos, D. G. (2002) Changing indications of open stone surgery. *Urology* 59: 490-493; discussion 493-494.

[36] Kaouk, J. H., Gill, I. S., Desai, M. M., Banks, K. L., Raja, S. S., et al. (2003) Laparoscopic anatrophic nephrolithotomy: feasibility study in a chronic porcine model. *J. Urol.* 169: 691-696.

[37] Assimos, D. G., Wrenn, J. J., Harrison, L. H., McCullough, D. L., Boyce, W. H., et al. (1991) A comparison of anatrophic nephrolithotomy and percutaneous nephrolithotomy with and without extracorporeal shock wave lithotripsy for management of patients with staghorn calculi. *J. Urol.* 145: 710-714.

[38] Esen, A. A., Kirkali, Z., Guler, C. (1994) Open stone surgery: is it still a preferable procedure in the management of staghorn calculi? *Int. Urol. Nephrol.* 26: 247-253.

[39] Goodwin, W. E., Casey, W. C., Woolf, W. (1955) Percutaneous trocar (needle) nephrostomy in hydronephrosis. *J. Am. Med. Assoc.* 157: 891-894.

[40] Dasgupta, P., Cynk, M. S., Bultitude, M. F., Tiptaft, R. C., Glass, J. M. (2004) Flexible ureterorenoscopy: prospective analysis of the Guy's experience. *Annals of the Royal College of Surgeons of England* 86: 367-370.

[41] Hunter, P. T., Finlayson, B., Drylie, D. M., Leal, J., Hawkins, I. F. (1985) Retrograde nephrostomy and percutaneous calculus removal in 30 patients. *The Journal of urology* 133: 369-374.

[42] Lawson, R. K., Murphy, J. B., Taylor, A. J., Jacobs, S. C. (1983) Retrograde method for percutaneous access to kidney. *Urology* 22: 580-582.

[43] Hawkins, I. F., Jr., Hunter, P., Leal, G., Nanni, G., Hawkins, M., et al. (1984) Retrograde nephrostomy for stone removal: combined cystoscopic/percutaneous technique. *AJR American journal of roentgenology* 143: 299-304.

[44] Kawahara, T., Ito, H., Terao, H., Kato, Y., Ogawa, T., et al. (2012) Ureteroscopy-Assisted Retrograde Nephrostomy (UARN) after Anatrophic Nephrolithotomy. *Case Rep. Med.* 2012: 164963.

[45] Wakeley, C. P. (1915) A Case of Duplication of the Ureters. *J. Anat. Physiol.* 49: 148-154.

[46] Inamoto, K., Tanaka, S., Takemura, K., Ikoma, F. (1983) Duplication of the renal pelvis and ureter: associated anomalies and pathological conditions. *Radiat. Med.* 1: 55-64.

[47] Ahmed, S., Pope, R. (1986) Uncrossed complete ureteral duplication with upper system reflux. *J. Urol.* 135: 128-129.

[48] Kawahara, T., Ito, H., Terao, H., Kato, Y., Ogawa, T., et al. (2012) Ureteroscopy-assisted retrograde nephrostomy (UARN) for an incomplete double ureter. *Urol. Res.* 40: 781-782.

[49] Raj, G. V., Auge, B. K., Weizer, A. Z., Denstedt, J. D., Watterson, J. D., et al. (2003) Percutaneous management of calculi within horseshoe kidneys. *J. Urol.* 170: 48-51.

[50] Osther, P. J., Razvi, H., Liatsikos, E., Averch, T., Crisci, A., et al. (2011) Percutaneous Nephrolithotomy Among Patients with Renal Anomalies: Patient Characteristics and Outcomes; a Subgroup Analysis of the Clinical Research Office of the Endourological Society Global Percutaneous Nephrolithotomy Study. *J. Endourol.*

[51] El Ghoneimy, M. N., Kodera, A. S., Emran, A. M., Orban, T. Z., Shaban, A. M., et al. (2009) Percutaneous nephrolithotomy in horseshoe kidneys: is rigid nephroscopy sufficient tool for complete clearance? A case series study. *BMC Urol.* 9: 17.

[52] Andreoni, C., Portis, A. J., Clayman, R. V. (2000) Retrograde renal pelvic access sheath to facilitate flexible ureteroscopic lithotripsy for the treatment of urolithiasis in a horseshoe kidney. *J. Urol.* 164: 1290-1291.

[53] Esuvaranathan, K., Tan, E. C., Tung, K. H., Foo, K. T. (1991) Stones in horseshoe kidneys: results of treatment by extracorporeal shock wave lithotripsy and endourology. *J. Urol.* 146: 1213-1215.

[54] Al-Otaibi, K., Hosking, D. H. (1999) Percutaneous stone removal in horseshoe kidneys. *J. Urol.* 162: 674-677.

[55] Jones, D. J., Wickham, J. E., Kellett, M. J. (1991) Percutaneous nephrolithotomy for calculi in horseshoe kidneys. *J. Urol.* 145: 481-483.

[56] Salas, M., Gelet, A., Martin, X., Sanseverino, R., Viguier, J. L., et al. (1992) Horseshoe kidney: the impact of percutaneous surgery. *Eur. Urol.* 21: 134-137.

[57] Stening, S. G., Bourne, S. (1998) Supracostal percutaneous nephrolithotomy for upper pole caliceal calculi. *J. Endourol.* 12: 359-362.

[58] De la Rosette, J., Assimos, D., Desai, M., Gutierrez, J., Lingeman, J., et al. (2011) The Clinical Research Office of the Endourological Society Percutaneous Nephrolithotomy Global Study: indications, complications, and outcomes in 5803 patients. *J. Endourol.* 25: 11-17.

[59] Kawahara, T., Ito, H., Terao, H., Tanaka, K., Ogawa, T., et al. (2012) Ureteroscopy-assisted retrograde nephrostomy for lower calyx calculi in horseshoe kidney: two case reports. *J. Med. Case Rep.* 6: 194.

[60] Ganpule, A. P., Desai, M. (2008) Management of the staghorn calculus: multiple-tract versus single-tract percutaneous nephrolithotomy. *Curr. Opin. Urol.* 18: 220-223.

[61] Preminger, G. M., Assimos, D. G., Lingeman, J. E., Nakada, S. Y., Pearle, M. S., et al. (2005) Chapter 1: AUA guideline on management of staghorn calculi: diagnosis and treatment recommendations. *J. Urol.* 173: 1991-2000.

[62] Kawahara, T., Ito, H., Terao, H., Yoshida, M., Ogawa, T., et al. (2011) Ureteroscopy assisted retrograde nephrostomy: a new technique for percutaneous nephrolithotomy (PCNL). *BJU Int.*

[63] Zimskind, P. D., Fetter, T. R., Wilkerson, J. L. (1967) Clinical use of long-term indwelling silicone rubber ureteral splints inserted cystoscopically. *The Journal of urology* 97: 840-844.

[64] Borboroglu, P. G., Kane, C. J. (2000) Current management of severely encrusted ureteral stents with a large associated stone burden. *The Journal of urology* 164: 648-650.

[65] Auge, B. K., Pietrow, P. K., Lallas, C. D., Raj, G. V., Santa-Cruz, R. W., et al. (2004) Ureteral access sheath provides protection against elevated

renal pressures during routine flexible ureteroscopic stone manipulation. *J. Endourol.* 18: 33-36.

[66]   Kawahara, T., Ito, H., Terao, H., Yoshida, M., Matsuzaki, J. (2011) Ureteral Stent Encrustation, Incrustation, and Coloring: Morbidity Related to Indwelling Times. *J. Endourol.* 26: 178-182.

[67]   Ho, C. H., Huang, K. H., Chen, S. C., Pu, Y. S., Liu, S. P., et al. (2009) Choosing the ideal length of a double-pigtail ureteral stent according to body height: study based on a Chinese population. *Urologia internationalis* 83: 70-74.

[68]   Joshi, H. B., Stainthorpe, A., MacDonagh, R. P., Keeley, F. X., Jr., Timoney, A. G., et al. (2003) Indwelling ureteral stents: evaluation of symptoms, quality of life and utility. *The Journal of urology* 169: 1065-1069; discussion 1069.

[69]   Pollard, S. G., Macfarlane, R. (1988) Symptoms arising from Double-J ureteral stents. *The Journal of urology* 139: 37-38.

[70]   Kawahara, T., Ito, H., Terao, H., Yoshida, M., Ogawa, T., et al. (2012) Choosing an Appropriate Length of Loop Type Ureteral Stent Using Direct Ureteral Length Measurement. *Urol. Int.* 88: 48-53.

[71]   Bultitude, M. F., Tiptaft, R. C., Glass, J. M., Dasgupta, P. (2003) Management of encrusted ureteral stents impacted in upper tract. *Urology* 62: 622-626.

[72]   Mohan-Pillai, K., Keeley, F. X., Jr., Moussa, S. A., Smith, G., Tolley, D. A. (1999) Endourological management of severely encrusted ureteral stents. *Journal of endourology / Endourological Society* 13: 377-379.

[73]   Schulze, K. A., Wettlaufer, J. N., Oldani, G. (1985) Encrustation and stone formation: complication of indwelling ureteral stents. *Urology* 25: 616-619.

[74]   El-Faqih, S. R., Shamsuddin, A. B., Chakrabarti, A., Atassi, R., Kardar, A. H., et al. (1991) Polyurethane internal ureteral stents in treatment of stone patients: morbidity related to indwelling times. *The Journal of urology* 146: 1487-1491.

[75]   Kawahara, T., Ito, H., Terao, H., Yoshida, M., Matsuzaki, J. (2011) Ureteral Stent Encrustation, Incrustation, and Coloring: Morbidity Related to Indwelling Times. *J. Endourol.*

[76]   Xu, C., Tang, H., Gao, X., Yang, B., Sun, Y. (2009) Management of forgotten ureteral stents with holmium laser. *Lasers in medical science* 24: 140-143.

[77]   Okuda, H., Yamanaka, M., Kimura, T., Takeyama, M. (2009) [Case of multiple encrusted stones on the ureteral stent left for 7 years: the

efficacy of extracting the ureteral stent on transurethral lithotripsy]. *Nippon Hinyokika Gakkai Zasshi* 100: 635-639.

[78] Kawahara, T., Ito, H., Terao, H., Ogawa, T., Uemura, H., et al. (2012) Encrusted Ureteral Stent Retrieval Using Flexible Ureteroscopy with a Ho: YAG Laser. *Case Rep. Med.* 2012: 862539.

[79] Kawahara, T., Ishida, H., Kubota, Y., Matsuzaki, J. (2012) Ureteroscopic removal of forgotten ureteral stent. *BMJ Case Rep.* 2012.

[80] Kawahara, T., Ito, H., Terao, H., Yoshida, M., Matsuzaki, J. (2012) Ureteral stent encrustation, incrustation, and coloring: morbidity related to indwelling times. *J. Endourol.* 26: 178-182.

[81] Ho, C. H., Huang, K. H., Chen, S. C., Pu, Y. S., Liu, S. P., et al. (2009) Choosing the ideal length of a double-pigtail ureteral stent according to body height: study based on a Chinese population. *Urol. Int.* 83: 70-74.

[82] Joshi, H. B., Stainthorpe, A., MacDonagh, R. P., Keeley, F. X., Jr., Timoney, A. G., et al. (2003) Indwelling ureteral stents: evaluation of symptoms, quality of life and utility. *J. Urol.* 169: 1065-1069; discussion 1069.

[83] Pollard, S. G., Macfarlane, R. (1988) Symptoms arising from Double-J ureteral stents. *J. Urol.* 139: 37-38.

[84] Wills, M. I., Gilbert, H. W., Chadwick, D. J., Harrison, S. C. (1991) Which ureteric stent length? *British journal of urology* 68: 440.

[85] Pocock, R. D., Stower, M. J., Ferro, M. A., Smith, P. J., Gingell, J. C. (1986) Double J stents. A review of 100 patients. *British journal of urology* 58: 629-633.

[86] Chin, J. L., Denstedt, J. D. (1992) Retrieval of proximally migrated ureteral stents. *The Journal of urology* 148: 1205-1206.

[87] Slaton, J. W., Kropp, K. A. (1996) Proximal ureteral stent migration: an avoidable complication? *The Journal of urology* 155: 58-61.

[88] Paick, S. H., Park, H. K., Byun, S. S., Oh, S. J., Kim, H. H. (2005) Direct ureteric length measurement from intravenous pyelography: does height represent ureteric length? *Urological research* 33: 199-202.

[89] Shah, J., Kulkarni, R. P. (2005) Height does not predict ureteric length. *Clinical radiology* 60: 812-814.

[90] Kawahara, T., Ito, H., Terao, H., Yoshida, M., Ogawa, T., et al. (2012) Which is the best method to estimate the actual ureteral length in patients undergoing ureteral stent placement? *Int. J. Urol.* 19: 634-638.

[91] Lingeman, J. E., Preminger, G. M., Goldfischer, E. R., Krambeck, A. E. (2009) Assessing the impact of ureteral stent design on patient comfort. *The Journal of urology* 181: 2581-2587.

[92] Joshi, H. B., Chitale, S. V., Nagarajan, M., Irving, S. O., Browning, A. J., et al. (2005) A prospective randomized single-blind comparison of ureteral stents composed of firm and soft polymer. *The Journal of urology* 174: 2303-2306.

[93] Dellis, A., Joshi, H. B., Timoney, A. G., Keeley, F. X., Jr. (2010) Relief of stent related symptoms: review of engineering and pharmacological solutions. *J. Urol.* 184: 1267-1272.

[94] Dunn, M. D., Portis, A. J., Kahn, S. A., Yan, Y., Shalhav, A. L., et al. (2000) Clinical effectiveness of new stent design: randomized single-blind comparison of tail and double-pigtail stents. *J. Endourol.* 14: 195-202.

[95] Kawahara, T., Ito, H., Terao, H., Yamashita, Y., Tanaka, K., et al. (2012) Ureteral stent exchange under fluoroscopic guidance using the crochet hook technique in women. *Urol. Int.* 88: 322-325.

[96] Kawahara, T., Ito, H., Terao, H., Yamagishi, T., Ogawa, T., et al. (2012) Ureteral stent retrieval using the crochet hook technique in females. *PLoS One* 7: e29292.

[97] Takashi Kawahara, H. I., Hideyuki Terao, Manabu Kakizoe, Yoshitake Kato, Hiroji Uemura, Yoshinobu Kubota, Junichi Matsuzaki (2013) Early ureteral catheter removal after ureteroscopic lithotripsy using ureteral access sheath. *Urolithiasis* 41: 31-35.

In: Ureters: Anatomy, Physiology and Disorders   ISBN: 978-1-62808-874-8
Editors: R. A. Santucci and M. Chen   © 2013 Nova Science Publishers, Inc.

Chapter 4

Stents in the Management of Ureteric Obstruction

Andreas Bourdoumis, Stefanos Kachrilas
and Noor Buchholz
Endourology and Stone Services, Barts Health NHS Trust, London, UK

Abstract

Many great advances of endourology are the result of the progress of indwelling stent technology and expansion of uses and applications. Ureteric obstruction can be caused by a variety of pathologies, both benign and malignant. This chapter shall begin with a brief description of classification and causes of ureteric obstruction. Imaging options will be reviewed in detail as precise characterization of the nature of an obstruction is pivotal when planning treatment options. Stent treatment options will be discussed, outlining principles, pathophysiology, and indication. Various types of stents and techniques will be presented considering the latest evidence (RCTs and meta-analyses). Success rates and complications will also be discussed. In addition, we will focus on dealing with strictures in urinary diversions, i.e. ileal conduit and transplant kidneys. The chapter will conclude with future perspectives on stent development.

Introduction

Advances in technology have contributed to our better understanding of the urinary tract and the development of diagnostic and therapeutic options for the management of contemporary urological problems. This is especially true for the upper urinary tract and management of obstruction. Much has changed since the introduction of the double J pigtail configuration in 1978. Modifications in design and evolution of biomaterials have taken place in order to improve efficacy and durability, as well as minimize patient discomfort. Ureteric stents are inserted when there is need for temporary or permanent decompression of the upper tract and preservation of renal function. This may be achieved by the retrograde or antegrade (percutaneous) route. Most commonly used materials include PTFE, metal mesh and full metal-bodied stents. Excluding impacted ureteric stones, conditions most commonly treated with indwelling ureteric stents include ureteropelvic junction obstruction, retroperitoneal fibrosis, pelvic lipomatosis and ureteral strictures.

1. Ureteropelvic Junction Obstruction (UPJO)

Obstruction at the ureteropelvic junction may be a result of a congenitally narrow and aperistaltic ureteral segment at the corresponding area or due to the presence of kinks, fibrous bands or adhesions. The importance of the aberrant lower pole renal vessel has been debated of late, yet it still holds significance since it still often seen at time of pyeloplasty. Acquired forms stem from previous inflammation, urolithiasis, benign or malignant tumors, postoperative scarring or ischemia and constitute rare conditions. Primary UPJO has an incidence of about 1:1500 with a slight male predominance and a predilection for the left side. [1] Although primarily a pediatric condition, UPJ obstruction may not become apparent until later. Diuretic renography with diuretic is the investigation of choice for diagnosing obstruction because it provides quantitative data regarding differential renal function and obstruction, even in hydronephrotic renal units. Pyeloplasty, either open or laparoscopic, is well recognized and the gold standard for repair. Recurrent stenosis leading to further symptoms is a late complication, possibly due to dense scarring or local fibrosis. The role of ureteral stents is for symptomatic relief of newly diagnosed UPJO prior to and after pyeloplasty. [2]

Stents are also widely used in cases of primary treatment failure and in candidates for laser endopyelotomy. Indeed, a recent study by Acher et al. favors placement before the procedure as it seems to improve functional outcome. [3] On the other hand, a contemporary study on a pediatric population in China by Kim et al. [4] showed no significant differences in the resolution of hydronephrosis or overall postoperative complications between stented and nonstented groups during dismembered pyeloplasty, in keeping with previously published evidence. [5]

Another aspect of stenting in ureteropelvic junction obstruction is concomitant renal pelvic or ureteric lithiasis. There is good evidence, albeit in few reports, to support a metabolic element to lithiasis in UPJO, rather the result of urinary stasis and obstruction to flow. In the retrospective study by Hussman [6], about 76% of patients undergoing pyeloplasty and simultaneous stone removal presented with a metabolic abnormality for several known lithogenic substances. The incidence of this finding in these patients was similar to that found in idiopathic stone formers. This abnormality consisted of varying levels of hypercalciuria, hyperoxaluria, hyperuricosuria and hypocitraturia.

The same authors subsequently reviewed a paediatric population with similar characteristics in retrospect, and found a recurrence rate of 68% in long term follow-up, with comparable results as for the metabolic factors found in adults, further supporting the concept of an underlying metabolic pathology [7].

Although the reports are scant in the literature, a reasonable approach would be to offer definitive treatment to symptomatic patients, especially those with deteriorating renal function and/or recurrent pain or infections. Initial stenting should be followed by pyelolithotomy and pyeloplasty by one of the many available treatment modalities. Patients unfit for surgery may be candidates for periodic stent changes.

2. Retroperitoneal Fibrosis

Retroperitoneal fibrosis is an uncommon condition with an estimated incidence of 1.38 cases per 100,000 people. [8] It includes a spectrum of diseases that lead to extensive fibroinflammatory tissue throughout the retroperitoneum, surrounding the abdominal aorta and the iliac arteries. This process may envelop surrounding structures, most commonly the ureters.

The majority of cases are idiopathic, with other causes such as drug-related, radiation-induced and malignant fibrosis being less common. However, biopsy to exclude malignancy should be performed whenever the diagnosis is contemplated. This is usually performed percutaneously with ultrasound, CT or MRI guidance. [9] Treatment usually involves corticosteroids, with or without other immunomodulating medications, or tamoxifen. Complications such as acute renal failure secondary to periureteral or perivascular involvement require prompt surgical intervention that includes placement of ureteral stents, percutaneous nephrostomy tubes, ureterolysis, and vascular stenting or surgery. Life-long follow-up with CT and diuretic renogram is recommended as the disease assumes a relapsing form.

Ureteral stents are used for the urgent management of symptomatic patients and to preserve renal function by adequate drainage. According to a series by Ilie et al. [10] ureteric stents relieved obstruction on all patients initially, while Katz et al. [11] reported that stenting facilitated later ureterolysis. Heidenreich et al. [12] used stents or nephrostomy for primary drainage in all patients in his study while treating with immunosuppressive regimes. Only four patients (recurrence rate 8%) remained eventually with DJ stents after a follow up of up to 120. This suggests that the best results come from a combination of medical and surgical treatment.

Ureterolysis is undertaken if medical therapy is contraindicated or fails to improve obstruction. Again, stents are used post operatively and can be removed 6 to 8 weeks after the procedure. [14] Success rates range 66% to 100% in various studies. [13-15] Chronic stenting is one alternative for situations where ureterolysis is technically challenging or fails. [14, 15] There is growing evidence that a combination of medical and surgical management carries the best overall success rate for the disease, with estimated recurrence rates between 5-8% in most series. [9, 12, 16] Periureteral involvement and/or progressive renal failure and uremia are the usual indications for surgical management.

3. Pelvic Lipomatosis

Pelvic lipomatosis is a rare, benign condition marked by overgrowth of nonmalignant but infiltrative adipose tissue, usually occurring in the perivesical and perirectal spaces. Engels first described the condition in 1959 and its etiology remains unknown to date. Links with obesity and a mutation in chromatin-regulating proteins have been made.

It tends to affect the male gender predominantly (male-to-female ratio: 18:1), yet the incidence is unknown. [17]

Klein et al. [18] suggested that there are two clinically separate groups of patients. The first is composed of young, stocky men with irritative lower urinary tract symptoms, vague pelvic complaints, hypertension, and proliferative cystitis. This group may be more susceptible to developing progressive ureteral obstruction.

The second group includes older men with incidentally discovered pelvic lipomatosis who have a more indolent course.

Progressive uremia may be found in up to 40% of patients. Surgical options in obstructive uropathy include ureteral stenting, percutaneous nephrostomy, ureteral reimplantation, and urinary diversion with or without cystoprostatectomy. [19]

4. Ureteric Strictures

4.1. Ureteric Stricture by Etiology

The classification of ureteric strictures may vary, subject to location, length and inciting factor. We have developed a novel system of characterizing a stricture, by distinguishing between primary and secondary elements that govern management.

As such, the nature of the stricture (benign versus malignant) and the involvement of the ureteric lumen (extrinsic versus intrinsic) are considered the primary elements (Figure 1). Stricture location, length, side, severity, etiology, and previous failed treatments are elements that play a role in further management.

Common causes of benign ureteric strictures include pelvic and retroperitoneal malignancy, ureteric lithiasis, prior radiation, iatrogenic injury, traumatic injury, periureteric fibrosis due to AAA, endometriosis or retroperitoneal fibrosis, and infection.

The obstruction may be a result of extrinsic compression or infiltration most commonly due to malignancy; intrinsic stenosis may be cause by instrumentation, urolithiasis and radiation treatment. Strictures developing in ureteroenteric anastomoses and ureteral reimplants of renal transplants merit special consideration due to the technical difficulties that are frequently encountered in the endourologic management of such patients.

Benign	Malignant
Ureteric Lithiasis	Urologic malignancy
Iatrogenic (instrumentation)	TCC Bladder / Ureter, Prostatic cancer
Traumatic (High velocity injury)	Gynecologic malignancy
Post-Radiation treatment	Cervical/Endometrial carcinoma
Post-Chemotherapy	
Infectious	
Endometriosis	
Retroperitoneal Fibrosis	
Ureteroileal anastomosis	
Idiopathic	

Extrinsic compression/ Benign Stricture	Extrinsic compression/ Malignant Stricture	Intrinsic compression/ Benign Stricture	Intrinsic compression/ Malignant Stricture
Idiopathic Retroperitoneal fibrosis	Gynecologic cancer (Cervix/Uterine)	Infectious (Tuberculosis, Schistosomiasis)	Transitional cell carcinoma of the ureter
Endometriosis	Colorectal cancer	Iatrogenic/Traumatic	Invasion by pelvic malignancy (i.e. prostate/ urinary bladder cancer)
	Cancer-related lymphadenopathy	Ureterointestinal anastomosis	
	Primary/Secondary Retroperitoneal malignancy	Post Renal Transplantation	
		Post-Radiation / Chemotherapy	
		Ureteric Lithiasis	

Figure 1. Ureteric stricture classification according to nature and luminal involvement.

4.1.1. Double J Stent or Percutaneous Nephrostomy?

The development and subsequent widespread use of the double J stent since 1978 has revolutionized the treatment of obstructive uropathy due to ureteric stricture, whether of benign or malignant cause. The question of retrograde stenting versus percutaneous nephrostomy as initial management of obstruction remains unanswered to this day. Modifications in design and evolution of biomaterials have taken place in order to improve efficacy and durability, as well as minimize patient discomfort. Ureteric stents are inserted when there is need for temporary or permanent decompression of the upper tract and preservation of renal function. This may be achieved by the retrograde or antegrade (percutaneous) route. Most commonly used materials include PTFE, metal mesh and full metal-bodied stents.

Practices vary greatly, although evidence exists now that percutaneous drainage is to be preferred upon impending sepsis, whereas retrograde stenting of the upper tracts may be chosen for uncomplicated cases and in coagulopathy. [20]

Several technical difficulties and specific patient characteristics pertaining to quality of life issue may influence the decision of primary management. For example, inability to identify the ureteral orifices or severe cardiopulmonary compromise may significantly compromise the outcome of either method. The availability of an experienced interventional radiology team is another factor when planning for future antegrade stenting post nephrostomy placement. Complication rate, albeit small, is an additional issue, especially for the elderly or frail patient. But perhaps the most crucial question to be answered is the real-life, contemporary benefit and long-term outcome of drainage for the given patient. Recent advances in guidewire and stent design, biocompatibility, and stenting technique have led to significant improvement in results. Success rate of retrograde stenting of 75% to 88% has been reported for both extrinsic [21-23] and intrinsic [24, 25] obstruction.

However, extrinsic malignant ureteral obstruction managed by double J stents has been associated with a high failure rate and significant morbidity in long term follow-up. One of the reasons for the failure is that the lumen occludes early by urinary debris or crystals and compression of the tumor prevents peri-stent drainage. Double J stents rely mainly on flow around the stent for drainage and less on intraluminal flow. [26, 27] Hyperplastic reaction, tumor ingrowth, encrustation and migration are principal reasons for compromised patency, making additional intervention necessary. The presence of mild urothelial hyperplasia with or without a trumpet-like configuration around the proximal stent edge is common and does not compromise ureteral patency significantly. Tumor ingrowth, on the other hand, is associated with obstruction and renal insufficiency. [28]

The difference in success rates may be related to the type of pelvic malignancy. Obstruction by bladder, prostatic or cervical malignancy managed in retrograde fashion presented with a success rate of only 15% to 21% compared to colorectal and breast cancer. [27] Regarding quality of life in patients with indwelling stents, irritative urinary symptoms seem to predominate. Febrile urinary tract infection has been reported in up to 10% of patients following double J stent insertion. [30] It has also been shown that stent length is an important factor for urinary symptoms, especially if the coil crosses at the midline. The same is true of placement of the proximal coil with adverse symptoms associated with placement outside the renal pelvis. [31]

Decompression by percutaneous nephrostomy (PCN) is a recognized method of improving renal function. [32, 33] However, the impact on the already depressed quality of life (QOL) of these patients is significant. [34, 35] Despite excellent drainage and no need for general anesthetic, a urine collection bag is required and complications such as bleeding, dislodgement, urosepsis, bowel and pleural injury can all be encountered when inserting a nephrostomy. In a recent report, up to one in five patients experienced pyelonephritis post PCN placement. [36] Furthermore, nephrostomy tube placement has not been shown to significantly prolong survival in patients with advanced cancer. One study demonstrated that only 11 of 17 patients with a PCN had acceptable QOL for 2 months or more. [37] Other problems that can contribute to poor QOL after PCN placement are urinary leakage and skin excoriation at the nephrostomy exit site. [39]

In an attempt to optimize management of obstruction, a staged approach may be desirable, in which a nephrostomy tube is initially placed using sedation and local anesthesia; 1-2 weeks after, an antegrade ureteral stent is placed. In that way, patients may be spared the complications of acute renal failure and/or hemodialysis and may also be relieved of intractable flank pain. In one such series, 59 of 60 patients were able to overcome ureteral obstruction with 57 of 60 successful after the first attempt at antegrade stenting. [40] Further studies are necessary to assess the usefulness of this procedure in patients with advanced malignant ureteral obstruction.

A summary of the principal studies on initial retrograde stenting for ureteric stricture according to site and initiating cause is depicted on Figure 2.

4.1.2. Metal Stents

Nitinol alloy is the latest metallic material used in ureteric stents and has enjoyed considerable success owing to its inherent shape memory and elasticity. It has paved the way for the development of full metal stents as the next step in stent design. The most widely studied and used metal stents include the Resonance® stent, the Memokath® stent, the Allium stent and the recently introduced Uventa® stent.

The Resonance® stent (Cook Ireland, Limerick, Ireland) is made of a nickel-cobalt-chromium-molybdenum alloy without a lumen. Urine flows through a spiral groove fashioned along the entire length of the stent. It is 6 Fr in caliber and is used mainly for extrinsic compression with a recommended indwelling time of 12 months. Liatsikos et al. reported 100% stricture patency rate in extraluminal malignant obstruction managed with Resonance stents and only 44% in benign strictures.

Study	No of patients	Type of stent used	Level of Obstruction	Patency rate (%)	Mean Follow-up (months)
Extrinsic Benign					
Rosevear et al[39] (2007)	8	Double J stent	Variable	100	16
Chung et al[26] (2004)	8	Double J stent	Proximal/Distal	88	11
Extrinsic Malignant					
Richter et al[40] (2000)	31	Wallstent	Lower ureter	58	42
Yossepowitch et al[41] (2001)	92	Double J stent	Variable	56.4	3
Chung et al[26] (2004)	100	Double J stent	Proximal/Distal	60	11
Ku et al[29] (2004)	68	Double J stent	Variable	89	9.2
Ganatra et al[27] (2005)	157	Double J stent	Variable	64.3	13.6
Rosevear et al[39] (2007)	29	Double J stent	Variable	81	16
Intrinsic Benign					
Wenzler et al[24] (2008)	38	Double J stent	Variable	88	25.5
Tal et al[25] (2007)	28	Double J stent	Ureterointestinal, Distal	45	62.5
Mallikarjuna et al,[42] (2006)	2	Metal mesh biliary	Lower ureter	100	18
Slavis et al,[43] (2000)	3	Wallstent	Mid ureter	100	51
Herrero et al,[44] (1996)	2	Wallstent	Transplant, Mid/Upper	100	18
Reinberg et al,[245] (1994)	3	Wallstent	Ureterointestinal, Distal	100	12
Intrinsic Malignant					
Danilovic et al,[46] (2005)	1	Double J stent	Proximal	100	NA

Figure 2. The most important studies for initial management of ureteric strictures with endoluminal stents.

Amongst complications, encrustation was found in 22% at the time of exchange. Obstruction, migration and stent related symptoms were also reported. Mean follow-up of the study was 8.5 months. [47] In a recent retrospective series of 19 patients by Wanq et al., the stricture patency rate was 77.3% for a mean follow-up of 5 months. Previous radiation therapy was identified as a risk factor for stent failure for malignant ureteral obstruction. [48] The Memokath 051® stent (Engineers and Doctors A/S, Copenhagen, Denmark) is a thermoexpandable shape memory stent made of nitinol with a lumen. It is introduced as a rigid cylinder which requires injection of sterile water at a temperature of 60 degrees Celcius in order to expand and shape it into the desirable position. For removal, it needs injection of cold water at 5 degrees Celcius to uncoil it prior to its removal. It is recommended for long term use in both intrinsic and extrinsic obstruction. Its segmental structure avoids lower urinary tract symptoms and reflux. It was first described by Kulkarni and Bellamy [49, 50] in 1999, with early follow-up showing no patient rehospitalizations for stent-related sepsis, pain, or hematuria. The 11-year follow-up data on 74 patients showed an overall stent migration rate of 18% and 19% reinsertion rate at a mean time of 7.1 months, of which only 3 were for stricture progression. Of the 28 patients with malignant obstruction, 89% (25/28) had post-procedural imaging showing normal or improved functional drainage. [51] In a recent study by Zaman et al., results were reported for 37 patients (mean age 64 years) suffering from malignant ureteric strictures. The mean follow-up was 22 months (range 5-60 months). Stent migration was reported in 13.5% (5 of 37), urinary tract infections in 8% (3 of 37) and blockage of stent due to progressive transitional cell carcinoma of the ureter in 5.4% (2 of 37) of cases. [52]

The Allium stent (Allium LTD, Caesarea, Israel) is the best studied representative of the group. It is a nickel titanium alloy mesh covered with a biocompatible polymer to prevent tissue ingrowth and encrustation. Patency rates are high (>95%), but followup in recent series do not exceed 24 months. Disadvantages of this stent include the requirement for initial ureteric balloon dilation and the difficult with stent adjustment in situ. [53] In addition, the design allows for use only in distal (VUJ) or proximal (PUJ) strictures. A full length Allium stent is currently in production and clinical trials awaited.

The Uventa® stent (TaeWoong Medical Co., LTD, Gveonggi-Do, Korea) incorporates a layer of PTFE between two super-elastic nitinol layers (triple layer) in a new expandable mesh, capable of treating the entire length of the ureter. Preliminary results are very promising with patency rates of 100% and minimal complications at a mean 7 months followup. [54]

Conclusion

Distinct gross and microscopic pathologic changes may occur with obstruction of the upper urinary tract. These may be affected by the presence of infection, duration of obstruction, and intra- versus extra-renal localization of the renal pelvis. A plethora of intraperitoneal and extraperitoneal disease processes may ultimately result in ureteral obstruction. Hydronephrosis, either symptomatic or incidental, may thus be the initial presentation of these conditions.

Drainage of the obstructed system is the first step in management in cases of threatened functional impairment or infection. Definitive management of the underlying pathology may then be considered as dictated by the disease process.

References

[1]   Smith, K. E. et al.: Stented versus nonstented pediatric pyeloplasty: A modern series and review of the literature. *J. Urol.* 2002;168:1127.

[2]   Plata, A. L., Faerber, G. J., Wolf, J. S. Jr. Stent placement for the diagnosis of upper tract obstruction. *Tech. Urol.* 1999 Dec.;5(4):207-9.

[3]   Acher, P. L., Nair, R., Abburaju, J. S., Dickinson, I. K., Vohra, A., Sriprasad, S. Ureteroscopic holmium laser endopyelotomy for ureteropelvic junction stenosis after pyeloplasty. *J. Endourol.* 2009 Jun.; 23(6):899-902.

[4]   Kim, J., Park, S., Hwang, H., Kim, J. W., Cheon, S. H., Park, S., Kim, K. S. Comparison of Surgical Outcomes between Dismembered Pyeloplasty with or without Ureteral Stenting in Children with Ureteropelvic Junction Obstruction. *Korean J. Urol.* 2012 Aug.;53(8): 564-8.

[5]   Smith, K. E., Holmes, N., Lieb, J. I., Mandell, J., Baskin, L. S., Kogan, B. A., Walker, R. D. 3rd. Stented versus nonstented pediatric pyeloplasty: a modern series and review of the literature. *J. Urol.* 2002 Sep.;168(3):1127-30.

[6]   Husmann, D. A., Milliner, D. S., Segura, J. W. Ureteropelvic junction obstruction with a simultaneous renal calculus: long-term follow up. *J. Urol.* 1995 May;153(5):1399-402.

[7] Husmann, D. A., Milliner, D. S., Segura, J. W. Ureteropelvic junction obstruction with concurrent renal pelvic calculi in the paediatric patient: a long-term follow up. *J. Urol.* 1996; 156:741-3.

[8] Van Bommel, E. F., Jansen, I., Hendriksz, T. R., Aarnoudse, A. L. Idiopathic retroperitoneal fibrosis: prospective evaluation of incidence and clinicoradiologic presentation. *Medicine* (Baltimore). 2009;88(4): 193-201.

[9] Baker, L. R., Mallinson, W. J., Gregory, M. C., Menzies, E. A., Cattell, W. R., Whitfield, H. N., Hendry, W. F., Wickham, J. E., Joekes, A. M. Idiopathic retroperitoneal fibrosis. A retrospective analysis of 60 cases. *Br. J. Urol.* 1987 Dec.;60(6):497-503.

[10] Ilie, C. P., Pemberton, R. J., Tolley, D. A. Idiopathic retroperitoneal fibrosis: the case for nonsurgical treatment. *BJU Int.* 2006 Jul.;98(1): 137-40

[11] Katz, R., Golijanin, D., Pode, D., Shapiro, A. Primary and postoperative retroperitoneal fibrosis-experience with 18 cases. *Urology.* 2002 Nov.;60 (5):780.

[12] Heidenreich, A., Derakhshani, P., Neubauer, S., Krug, B. Treatment outcomes in primary and secondary retroperitoneal fibrosis. *Urologe A.* 2000 Mar.;39(2):141-8.

[13] Elashry, O. M., Nakada, S. Y., Wolf, J. S. Jr, et al. Ureterolysis for extrinsic ureteral obstruction: a comparison of laparoscopic and open surgical techniques. *J. Urol.* 1996 Oct.;156(4):1403-10.

[14] Fugita, O. E., Jarrett, T. W., Kavoussi, P., et al. Laparoscopic treatment of retroperitoneal fibrosis. *J. Endourol.* 2002 Oct.;16(8):571-4.

[15] Duchene, D. A., Winfield, H. N., Cadeddu, J. A., et al. Multi-institutional survey of laparoscopic ureterolysis for retroperitoneal fibrosis. *Urology.* 2007 Jun.;69(6):1017-21.

[16] Kermani, T. A., Crowson, C. S., Achenbach, S. J., Luthra, H. S. Idiopathic retroperitoneal fibrosis: a retrospective review of clinical presentation, treatment, and outcomes. *Mayo. Clin. Proc.* 2011 Apr.;86 (4):297-303.

[17] Heyns, C. F. Pelvic lipomatosis: a review of its diagnosis and management. *J. Urol.* 1991 Aug.;146(2):267-73.

[18] Klein, F. A., Smith, M. J., Kasenetz, I. Pelvic lipomatosis: 35-year experience. *J. Urol.* 1988 May;139(5):998-100.

[19] Sözen, S., Gürocak, S., Uzüm, N., et al. The importance of re-evaluation in patients with cystitis glandularis associated with pelvic lipomatosis: a case report. *Urol. Oncol.* 2004 Sep.-Oct.;22(5):428-30.

[20] Lynch, M. F., Anson, K. M., Patel, U. Percutaneous nephrostomy and ureteric stent insertion for acute renal deobstruction. Consensus based guidelines. *Br. J. Med. Surg. Urol.* 2008 Nov.;1(3);120-5.

[21] Radecka, E., Magnusson, M. and Magnusson, A.: Survival time and period of catheterization in patients treated with percutaneous nephrostomy for urinary obstruction due to malignancy. *Acta Radiol.* 2006; 47: 328.

[22] Chapman, M. E. and Reid, J. H.: Use of percutaneous nephrostomy in malignant ureteric obstruction. *Br. J. Radiol.* 1991; 64: 318.

[23] Rosenberg, B. H., Bianco, F. J. Jr, Wood, D. P. Jr, Triest, J. A. Stent-change therapy in advanced malignancies with ureteral obstruction. *J. Endourol.* 2005 Jan.-Feb.;19(1):63-7.

[24] Wenzler, D. L., Kim, S. P., Rosevear, H. M., Faerber, G. J., Roberts, W. W., Wolf, J. S. Jr. Success of ureteral stents for intrinsic ureteral obstruction. J. Endourol. 2008 Feb.;22(2):295-9.

[25] Tal, R., Sivan, B., Kedar, D., Baniel, J. Management of benign ureteral strictures following radical cystectomy and urinary diversion for bladder cancer. *J. Urol.* 2007 Aug.;178(2):538-42.

[26] Chung, S. Y., Stein, R. J., Landsittel, D., et al.: 15-Year experience with the management of extrinsic ureteral obstruction with indwelling ureteral stents. *J. Urol.* 2004; 172: 592.

[27] Ganatra, A. M. and Loughling, K. M.: The management of malignant ureteral obstruction treated with ureteral stents. *J. Urol.* 2006; 174: 2125.

[28] Kouba, E., Wallen, E. M., Pruthi, R. S. Management of ureteral obstruction due to advanced malignancy: optimizing therapeutic and palliative outcomes. *J. Urol.* 2008 Aug.;180(2):444-50.

[29] Ku, J. H., Lee, S. W., Jeon, H. G., Kim, H. H., and Oh, S. J.: Percutaneous nephrostomy versus indwelling ureteral stents in the management of extrinsic ureteral obstruction in advanced malignancies: are there differences? *Urology* 2004; 64: 895.

[30] El-Nahas, A. R., El-Assmy, A. M., Shoma, A. M., Eraky, I., El-Kenawy, M. R., and El-Kappany, H. A.: Self-retaining ureteral stents: analysis of factors responsible for patients' discomfort. *J. Endourol.* 2006; 20: 33.

[31] Pappas, P., Stravodimos, K. G., Mitropoulos, D., et al. Role of percutaneous urinary diversion in malignant and benignobstructive uropathy. *J. Endourol.* 2000;14:401–405

[32] Carrafiello, G., Lagana, D., Lumia, D., et al. Direct primary or secondary percutaneous ureteral stenting: What is the most compliant

option in patients with malignant ureteral obstructions? *Cardiovasc. Intervent. Radiol.* 2007;30:974–980.

[33]   Aravantinos, E., Anagnostou, T., Karantzas, A. D., et al.: Percutaneous nephrostomy in patients with tumors of advanced stage: treatment dilemmas and impact on clinical course and quality of life. *J. Endourol.* 2007; 21: 1297.

[34]   Joshi, H. B., Adams, S., Obadeyi, O. O., Rao, P. N. Nephrostomy tube or 'JJ' ureteric stent in ureteric obstruction: assessment of patient perspectives using quality-of-life survey and utility analysis. *Eur. Urol.* 2001 Jun.;39(6):695-701.

[35]   Bahu, R., Chaftari, A., Hachem, R. Y., et al. Nephrostomy Tube Related Pyelonephritis in Patients with Cancer: Epidemiology, Infection Rate and Risk Factors. *J. Urol.* 2013 Vol. 189, 130-135.

[36]   Emmert, C., Rassler, J. and Kohler, U.: Survival and quality of life after percutaneous nephrostomy for malignant ureteric obstruction in patients with terminal cervical cancer. *Arch. Gynecol. Obstet.* 1997; 259: 147.

[37]   Schmidbauer, J., Kratzik, C., Klingler, H. C., Remzi, M., Lackner, J., and Marberger, M.: Nephrovesical subcutaneous ureteric bypass: long-term results in patients with advanced metastatic disease—improvement of renal function and quality of life. *Eur. Urol.* 2006; 50: 1073.

[38]   Chitale, S. V., Scott-Barrett, S., Ho, E. T., and Burgess, N. A.: The management of ureteric obstruction secondary to malignant pelvic disease. *Clin. Radiol.* 2002; 57: 1118.

[39]   Rosevear, H. M., Kim, S. P., Wenzler, D. L., et al. Retrograde ureteral stents for extrinsic ureteral obstruction: nine years' experience at University of Michigan. *Urology.* 2007 Nov.;70(5):846-50.

[40]   Richter, F., Irwin, R. J., Watson, R., Lang, E. Endourologic management of malignant ureteral strictures. *J. Endourol.* 2000; 14:583–587.

[41]   Yossepowitch, O., Lifshitz, D. A., Dekel, Y.,et al. Predicting the success of retrograde stenting for managing ureteral obstruction. *J. Urol.* 2001 Nov.;166(5):1746-9

[42]   Mallikarjuna, C., Suri Babu, A., Vijaya Kumar, K. UP-01.06: Permanent metallic stents in ureteric strictures.*Urology* 68 (Supplement 5A), November 2006

[43]   Slavis, S. A., Wilson, R., Jones, R., Swift, C. Long-Term Results of Permanent Indwelling Wallstents for Benign Mid-ureteral Strictures. *J. Endourol.* 2000; 14 (7):577-81.

[44] Herrero, J. A., Lezana, A., Gallego, J., et al. Self-expanding metallic stent in the treatment of ureteral obstruction after renal transplantation. *Nephrol. Dial. Transplant* 1996;11:887.

[45] Reinberg, Y., Ferral, H., Gonzalez, R., Manivel, J. C., Hulbert, J., Maynar, M., Pulido-Duque, J. M., Hunter, D., Castaneda-Zuniga, W. R. Intraureteral metallic self-expanding endoprosthesis (Wallstent) in the treatment of difficult ureteral strictures. *J. Urol.* 1994 Jun.;151(6):1619-22.

[46] Danilovic, A., Antonopoulos, I. M., Mesquita, J. L., Lucon, A. M. Likelihood of retrograde double-J stenting according to ureteral obstructing pathology. *Int. Braz. J. Urol.* 2005 Sep.-Oct.;31(5):431-6; discussion 436.

[47] Liatsikos, E., Kallidonis, P., Kyriazis, I., Constantinidis, C., Hendlin, K., Stolzenburg, J. U., et al. (2010) Ureteral obstruction: is the full metallic double-pigtail stent the way to go? *Eur. Urol.* 2010; 57: 480–487.

[48] Wang, H. J., Lee, T. Y., Luo, H. L., Chen, C. H., Shen, Y. C., Chuang, Y. C., Chiang, P. H. Application of resonance metallic stents for ureteral obstruction. *BJU Int.* 2011 Aug.;108(3):428-32.

[49] Kulkarni, R. P., Bellamy, E. A. A new thermo-expandable shapememory nickel-titanium alloy stent for the management of ureteric strictures. *BJU Int.* 1999;83:755–759.

[50] Kulkarni, R., Bellamy, E. Nickel-titanium shape memory alloy Memokath 051 ureteral stent for managing long-term ureteral obstruction: 4-year experience. *J. Urol.* 2001;166:1750–1754.

[51] Agrawal, S., Brown, C. T., Bellamy, E. A., Kulkarni, R. The thermoexpandable metallic ureteric stent: An 11-year follow-up. *BJU Int.* 2009;103:372–376.

[52] Zaman, F., Poullis, C., Bach, C., Moraitis, K., Junaid, I., Buchholz, N., Masood, J. Use of a segmental thermoexpandable metal alloy stent in the management of malignant ureteric obstruction: a single centre experience in the UK. *Urol. Int.* 2011;87(4):405-10.

[53] Moskovitz, B., Halachmi, S., Nativ, O. A New Self-Expanding, Large-Caliber Ureteral Stent: Results of a Multicenter Experience. *J. of Endourol.* 2012; 26 (11):1523–27.

[54] Kim, J. H., Song, K., Ki Jo, M., Park, J. W. Palliative Care of Malignant Ureteral Obstruction with Polytetrafluoroethylene Membrane-Covered Self-Expandable Metallic Stents: Initial Experience. *Korean J. Urol.* 2012 September; 53(9): 625–631

In: Ureters: Anatomy, Physiology and Disorders   ISBN: 978-1-62808-874-8
Editors: R. A. Santucci and M. Chen   © 2013 Nova Science Publishers, Inc.

Chapter 5

Metallic Stents for Malignant Upper Urinary Tract Obstruction

Petros Sountoulides[1,] and Anastasios Anastasiadis[2]*
[1]Urology Department, General Hospital of Veria, Greece
[2]1st Urology Department, Aristotle University of Thessaloniki,
Thessaloniki, Greece

Abstract

Upper urinary tract obstruction is an everyday situation for practicing urologists. The usual options for decompression of obstruction include the insertion of a double-J stent or the placement of a nephrostomy tube. However, the situation is getting more complicated when malignancy is the cause of upper tract obstruction. Causes for obstruction of the urinary tract related to malignancy include retroperitoneal lymphatic masses, post-radiation or chemotherapy strictures and advanced bladder or prostate cancer. Malignant upper tract obstruction requires long-term or even permanent solutions and is more difficult to manage compared to benign causes such as stones. Although the evolution of stents has provided a viable option for the management of the majority of causes of upper tract obstruction, malignant disease can be recalcitrant to routine

* Corresponding author: Petros Sountoulides, Address: 15-17 Agiou Evgeniou street, 55133, Thessaloniki, Greece. Phone: +30 6944696849; E-mail: sountp@hotmail.com.

stent placement. Stent migration, infection, calcification and obstruction are unfortunately common problems when stents are used in this setting.

For this reason metallic ureteral stents of different designs and materials have been adopted in the management of malignant upper tract obstruction with mixed results. This commentary aims to retrospect on the evolution of metallic stents and their outcomes in alleviating malignant ureteral obstruction and also provide some insights into the future of stent design and utilization in Urology.

Introduction

The main reason for placement of a ureteral stent is maintaining patency of the upper urinary tract in cases where this is compromised by acute or chronic, intrinsic or extrinsic, benign or malignant, obstruction. Toward this goal, a variety of configurations, designs, and materials have been utilized since the first introduction of a ureteral "stent" in urological practice by Gibbons back in 1976 (Gibbons 1976).

Still, it was not before the introduction of the double-J, or pigtail, stent by Finney that the use of ureteral stents was popularized (Finney 1978).

In the setting of malignant obstruction of the upper urinary tract, effective urinary drainage has been traditionally achieved by internal ureteral stenting or placement of a nephrostomy tube. And while stenting is preferred to nephrostomy by both patients and physicians (Chung 2004) it has proven to be far from uneventful.

The presence of stents in the ureter has been associated with impeded flow of urine, hyperplastic reaction, stent encrustation, stent migration and infection as well as inability to successfully maintain patency of the upper urinary tract. Certain modifications in stent design, material and configuration have been proposed attempting at reducing the discomfort and reduced quality of life associated with the presence of indwelling plastic ureteral stents and the subsequent need for periodic stent changes.

The introduction of metallic stents has provided solutions to some of the limitations of conventional stents and revolutionized the management of upper tract obstruction caused by malignancy. This commentary will briefly discuss the evolution of metallic stents over time; present their current outcomes and point towards future directions.

Aetiology and Management of Malignant Upper Tract Obstruction

Bilateral or unilateral malignant ureteral obstruction may be secondary to direct tumor invasion, extrinsic compression, or encasement of the ureter by metastatic retroperitoneal or pelvic lymph nodes. A primary retroperitoneal tumor arising near the ureter may result in local infiltration and obstruction of the ureter. Previous surgery or radiotherapy may also cause late stricture formation and subsequent upper tract obstruction (Yachia 2008, Harding 1995).

Upper tract decompression is required in order to restore renal function, alleviate pain, and resolve obstructive upper urinary tract infection. Uremia and resultant chronic kidney disease due to malignant ureteric obstruction is a well-described event in the course of advanced malignancy, usually of pelvic origin, which, if left untreated, may quickly become a terminal event. Prompt ureteral decompression is an important component in the treatment of these patients, as part of palliative or definitive management of the primary malignancy. Options for ureteral decompression include plastic ureteral stents, metal wall stents, full-length metal stents, nephrostomy drainage, ureteral dilation, ureterolysis, cutaneous ureterostomy, and temporary urinary diversion (Sountoulides, J Endourol 2010). Some of these options may, however, be precluded by the attendant surgical morbidity or history of radiation treatment (Okeke 2008).

Contemporary management options mainly involve external drainage via percutaneous nephrostomy (PCN) and internal drainage via the insertion of double-J stents. Decompression of the obstructed upper tract results in improved renal function, with presumed low morbidity, and better quality of life. However, PCN is considered more invasive than double-J stent placement and may also have a greater incidence of tube dislodgement. The invasiveness of the procedure and the high incidence of tube dislodgement may result in a deterioration in quality of life. In addition, some patients are unwilling to accept a PCN tube because it requires an external collecting device. The selection of cancer patients for diversion should take into account factors such as tumor stage, prognosis of the primary cancer, likelihood of additional antineoplastic therapy, and quality of life. The limitations associated with conventional treatments for ureteral obstructions highlight the need for a novel treatment that can maintain ureteral patency while minimizing the deterioration of patient quality of life (Wilson 2005, Kim 2012).

Efficacy and Limitations of Stents

Since patients presenting with malignant ureteric obstruction usually suffer from advanced malignancy, the procedures used for urinary diversion are generally palliative. Polyurethane and silicon stents are used because they are considered to be more inert in nature than metals or other substances. However, polymeric stents demonstrate certain limits in their ability to resist external compression forces (Ganatra 2006, Christmas 2009).

This shortcoming has been repeatedly corroborated by clinical experience showing a significant rate of stent failure ranging from 35 to 44% (Christmas, Chung). The most common malignancies causing ureteral obstruction were gynecologic and gastrointestinal in origin, and invasion of the bladder from prostate cancer was found to significantly increase the risk of stent failure (Ganatra 2006).

In the series reported by Chung, 90 patients underwent ureteral decompression for malignant ureteral obstruction. The investigators reported a 44% failure rate for stent placement within a mean follow-up time of 11 months. Of the patients in whom stent placement failed, only 27% elected to have nephrostomy tubes inserted (Chung 2004). In another series of 28 patients treated for malignant ureteral obstruction with ureteral stents reported by Rosenberg and associates, (Rosenberg 2005) only 3 of 28 patients ultimately experienced stent failure and needed nephrostomy tube drainage, although a total of 7 patients experienced worsening renal function despite ureteral stents. The most commonly reported complication was urinary tract infection, with 64% of patients experiencing at least one episode. While many of these patients had multiple hospital admissions, most were for complaints related to the underlying malignancy. Stent-related admissions were mainly because of urinary tract infections (Okeke 2008).

Metallic Stents: A Brief Overview of Evolution and Results

Metallic ureteral stents were introduced for the management of malignant upper tract obstruction in an attempt to overcome the problems of early stent obstruction, encrustation, tumor ingrowth and need for frequent stent changes. Stent exchange in patients with advanced malignancies can be the source of significant morbidity and mortality, as stent change can be technically difficult or even impossible. Stent changes might also require overnight hospitalization or anaesthesia - all of which are posing certain risks for patients with malignancies.

Therefore in the setting of malignant ureteral obstruction (MUO) there is a clear need for stents that can be left in situ for prolonged periods providing safe and efficient drainage of the upper urinary tract sparing the morbidity encountered with the regular stents. The theoretical advantages of metal stents over polymer ones included reduced encrustation, improved tensile strength and stability, prolonged stent indwell time, and better flow.

A variety of metallic alloys, designs, lengths and configurations of metallic ureteral stents have been used during the last decades. The *self–expandable elastic mesh stent* (Wallstent), made of stainless cobalt, was introduced in the early 90's for use in ureteral stenosis. However experience with its use was not encouraging mainly due to its low patency rates requiring additional procedures such as repeat balloon dilation and coaxial stenting. (Pauer 1992)

Thermo-expandable stents (Memokath) made from nickel-titanium alloy, initially used for the relief of lower urinary tract obstruction, were then also introduced in upper tract obstruction in an effort to overcome the problems of encrustation, urothelial hyperplasia and difficult removal that were common with the self-expandable stents. In theory the Memokath was ideal as it has shape-memory, a low propensity for encrustation and a tight spiral configuration designed to minimize tissue ingrowth.

In real life though, insertion or removal of a Memokath stent was not an easy task due to the need for precise estimation of the length and location of the stricture for correct stent placement.

Also placement and removal of such stents was not always uneventful, and often required a fully equipped endourological suite and high endourological skills. Stent migration and encrustation continued to be problematic, and soon the need for a better stent became a reality. (Sountoulides, BJUInt 2010)

In addition, the efficacy of bare self-expandable and balloon-expandable metal stents is limited by issues such as the hyperplastic ingrowth through the side-holes of the stents resulting in stent occlusion. A solution at that time was the introduction of *covered metal stents* using various biocompatible materials in an effort to prevent tissue ingrowth and minimize urothelial trauma. The rationale was that stents covered with various biocompatible materials in the absence of side-holes would limit the ingrowth of hyperplastic tissue into the ureteric lumen. Again, in clinical practice, initial results were not enthusiastic.

The Passager stent, a flexible stent externally covered with ultrathin woven polyester fabric, demonstrated a high failure rate mainly due to bladder migration following initial successful placement. Failure was attributed to increased ureteral peristalsis and stent migration due to inadequate stent adherence to the ureteral wall. (Barbalias, 2002)

Dacron nitinol covered stents have also been used for the management of MUO. Nitinol is a titanium-nickel shape memory alloy with biocompatibility, flexibility, radial strength, and compression resistance, considered easily adaptable to tortuous ureters. Dacron is an inert polyester with a smooth surface that does not permit fibrous tissue ingrowth. Overall, the initial experience with the Dacron-covered stents was encouraging (Tekin 2001).

A nitinol stent (Hemobahn Endoprosthesis, WL Gore and Associates, Newark, Delaware, US) completely covered with expanded PTFE, previously used for the management of obstructive biliary malignancies, has also been used for malignant upper tract obstruction (Bezzi 2002). The Hemobahn endoprothesis is internally covered by the PTFE so that the outer metallic mesh makes direct contact with the urothelium for better anchoring of the stent to the ureteric wall. Although the preliminary results were significantly better than those with the Passager stent, stent migration still occurred in 22% of cases and was resolved by the placement of a second stent (Trueba 2004).

At the end of the day, and despite certain advancements, all of the metal stents discussed previously share, to a greater or lesser extent, several drawbacks: a) they are short semi-permanent stents, b) they easily migrate due to their size and limited adherence to the ureteral wall, c) patency is not guaranteed and thus placement of additional stents or other anchillary procedures may be required. (Klarskov 2005, Liatsikos, J. Urol. 2009) The search for a better stent in order to manage MUO is thus ongoing. Ideally this stent should be easily placed and removed, should maintain upper tract patency despite extrinsic compression without additional interventions, and it should safely dwell for longer periods allowing for less frequent stent changes.

Coiled reinforced metallic stents, introduced in the late 00's were theoretically able to address all of the aforementioned issues. This category of coiled reinforced metallic stents initially included the Resonance® stent (Cook Urological, Indiana, US) and the Silhouette® stent (Applied Medical, Cleveland, US). One of the most important advantages of these stents was the improved resistance to extrinsic radial compression, a parameter that is important for preventing occlusion of the lumen due to tumor ingrowth or extrinsic stent compression.

Also the stents' low tensile strength, together with the appropriate selection of stent length, are important factors for preventing stent migration and patient discomfort (Miyaoka, 2010, Borin, 2006).

Both the Resonance and the Silhouette stents have been tested in vitro for tensile strength, stiffness, and resistance to compression compared with the C-Flex stent (Cook Medical, Indiana, US). Both coiled stents were less stiff than the C-Flex stent, while the Resonance stent demonstrated the higher tensile strength. The Silhouette stent was found to be the most resistant to extrinsic compression (Pedro, 2007).

The *Resonance*® *stent* is a 6F continuous non-fenestrated metal coil with an inner safety wire welded to both closed ends. It is constructed of MP35N® alloy, a composite of nonmagnetic nickel–cobalt–chromium–molybdenum with a unique combination of ultrahigh tensile strength and excellent resistance to corrosion. In contrast to the variety of short metal stents, the Resonance is designed in the style of an indwelling full-length ureteric stent with conventional pig-tail ends but no end-holes. For this reason this 6F stent cannot be passed over a guidewire, instead it is passed over an 8-10F introducer-dilator. Improved patency rates theoretically allow for a 1-year indwelling time before stent change.

As the Resonance stent has no end-holes, urine drainage is accomplished by a combination of extraluminal and intraluminal flow. In detail, urine drains primarily around the outer aspect of the spiral coiled metal; however, in cases of increased pressure within the upper tract, urine can enter the internal lumen of the coil (Blaschko 2007, Gamboa, 2008). The unique properties of the particular alloy of the Resonance stent should, in theory, prevent hyperplastic tissue ingrowth and encrustation, and improve the stent's biocompatibility. A recent study with the use of electron microscopy and spectroscopy has confirmed the lack of epithelial tissue ingrowths and durability of the Resonance® stent (Cauda 2010).

Although extensive *clinical experience* is still lacking, initial reports were highly favorable (Borin, 2006, Wah, 2007). Wah et al. reported their experience with the Resonance stent in a series of patients with malignant ureteral obstruction. Seventeen Resonance stents were antegradely placed in fifteen patients with various malignancies prior to adjuvant chemotherapy. Three of the seventeen stents had failed from the first day as was evident by nephrostograms and renal function deterioration.

All three stents were placed in patients with bulky pelvic disease and all of them were subsequently maintained on external drainage by percutaneous nephrostomies.

The rest of the stents were functioning properly with no evidence to suggest stent blockage during their follow-up period of every 6-12 months (time of stent change). Encrustation was minimal in all cases where the stents were changed after some months. Stents were easily changed cystoscopically by urologists (Wah, 2007).

Liatsikos et al. reviewed the outcomes of the Resonance stents with regard to technical success and patency rates in 25 patients within a reasonable follow up time (8.5 months) (Liatsikos, 2010). The success rate for stent placement was 100% and all stents remained patent during follow-up. Notably, the success and patency rates of the Resonance stents were significantly worse in cases of benign compared to malignant ureteral obstruction.

There is evidence that the Resonance® stent apart from maintaining upper tract patency is also more cost-effective in the long-term compared to the traditional double-J stents mainly due to their longer exchange intervals which could exceed 1 year according to the manufacturer (Lopez-Huertas, 2010, Polcari, 2010, Taylor, 2012).

While metallic stents have shown patency rates averaging greater than the 3 to 6 months typically seen with polymer stents, patients still need to be followed closely for evidence of obstruction, encrustation, infection or painful stent symptoms since there is no clear evidence of safety for recommending an optimal indwelling time (Modi, 2010). Cystoscopy can be a tool for monitoring stent encrustation as the visual appearance of encrustation at the distal end of a stent may correlate with upper stent encrustation. However, placement times need to be balanced with the likelihood of safe and efficient removal.

Recent studies with longer follow up have somewhat lessened the initial excitement about the efficacy of the Resonance stent. In the study from an academic referral center in Durham, from a total of 37 stents placed in 25 patients with malignant ureteral obstruction, 12 (35%) were identified to fail. Progressive hydroureteronephrosis and increasing creatinine were the most common signs of stent failure. Patients with evidence of prostate cancer invading the bladder at stent placement were found to have a significantly increased risk of failure. According to the authors' experience, the failure rates with metallic stents are similar to those historically observed with traditional polyurethane-based stents in malignant ureteral obstruction (Goldsmith, 2012). The same discouraging results were reached in the study by Gayed et al. in two of pediatric patients with extrinsic ureteral obstruction. The authors found the patency rates for the Resonance stents were much lower than those reported for adults (Gayed, 2013).

On the contrary, a Chinese retrospective study on 20 patients found the Resonance stent to demonstrate excellent patency rates in cases of both benign and malignant obstructions with the exception of radiotherapy patients (50% patency rate) (Li, 2011).

Although the results of current studies on the efficacy of the Resonance stent are mixed, (Rao, 2011) there is evidence that the Resonance stent holds promise for the effective management of patients with malignant obstruction of the upper urinary tract.

Stents of the (Near?) Future

Following the footsteps of the Resonance stent, a new generation of metallic stents is under way aiming at improving the clinical results accomplished with the coil-reinforced stents in relation to MUO. These new stent designs include the Passage™ (Prosurg Inc, California, US) 7F metallic coil stent and the Snake™ (Prosurg Inc, California, US) stents. The Passage stent, released in 2010, is a flexible metallic coil stent with a spiral winding configuration combining flexibility with durable radial compression strength. The Passage stent design with central lumen allows familiar retrograde cystoscopic insertion of the stent using the guidewire and pusher technique. The Snake gold-plated, metallic spring coiled ureteral stent has flexible pigtails and comes in two designs; one is 6F while the second is somewhat larger (7 F); its straight section is covered with biocompatible polymer tubing. In contrast to the Resonance stent, which is tightly coiled around a stainless steel guidewire and closed at both ends, these stents are less tightly wound and open at both ends.

These new stents have been recently tested in vitro for physical characteristics including coil strength, tensile strength and resistance to extrinsic compression. The Snake 6Fr stent was the one having the lowest tensile strength followed by the Passage and Snake 7F stents. The elastic modulus required to cause extrinsic compression was highest for the Snake 6Fr stent compared to that of the Passage and Snake 7F stents. A low tensile strength together with a high coil strength are important for prevention of stent migration while a high resistance to extrinsic radial compression is vital for preventing obstruction due to tumor ingrowth or extrinsic stent compression (Hendlin, 2012).

In addition, the authors found that the increase of stent diameter of 1Fr weakened the resistance of radial compression.

Therefore in situations where a metal stent is used for alleviation of ureteral obstruction, a 6Fr stent may be more effective in sustaining ureteral patency over a 7Fr stent where radial compression is the greatest threat (Liatsikos, 2005, 2010).

Conclusion

Relieving ureteral obstruction caused by malignancy is a demanding and challenging task for both physicians and patients alike. Proof of that is the constant evolution of stents fueled by increased patient and physician needs and expectations. Undoubtedly, management of malignant upper tract obstruction will continue to improve with stents that are easier to place, harder to occlude, and less bothersome to the patient.

References

Barbalias, G. A., Liatsikos, E. N., Kalogeropoulou, C., et al. Externally coated ureteral metallic stents: an unfavorable clinical experience. *Eur. Urol.* 2002; 42: 276–80

Bezzi, M., Zolovkins, A., Cantisani, V., et al. New ePTFE/FEP-covered stent in the palliative treatment of malignant biliary obstruction. *J. Vasc. Interv. Radiol.* 2002; 13: 581–9

Blaschko, S. D., Deane, L. E., Krebs, A., et al. In-vivo evaluation of flow characteristics of novel metal ureteral stent. *J. Endourol.* 2007; 21: 780–3

Borin, J. F., Melamud, O., Clayman, R. V. Initial experience with full-length metal stent to relieve malignant ureteral obstruction. *J. Endourol.* 2006; 20:300–304.

Cauda, V., Fiori, C., Cauda, F. Ni-Cr-Co alloy ureteral stent: Scanning electron microscopy and elemental analysis characterization after long-term indwelling. *J. Biomed. Mater. Res. B Appl. Biomater.* 2010;94:501-7.

Christman, M. S., L'esperance, J. O., Choe, C. H., Stroup, S. P., Auge, B. K. Analysis of ureteral stent compression force and its role in malignant obstruction. *J. Urol.* 2009;181:392–6.

Chung, S. Y., Stein, R. J., Landsittel, D., Davies, B. J., Cuellar, D. C., Hrebinko, R. L., Tarin, T., Averch, T. D. 15-year experience with the management of extrinsic ureteral obstruction with indwelling ureteral stents. *J. Urol.* 2004 Aug.;172(2):592-5.

Finney, R. P. Experience with a new double-J ureteral catheter stent. *J. Urol.* 1978;120:678-81.

Gamboa, A., Louie, M., Andrade, L., et al. Evaluation of Flow Characteristics in a Novel Metal Ureteric Stent (Resonance Stent) in a Porcine Model. *J. Endourol.* 2008; 22(s1):139.

Ganatra, A. M., Loughling, K. M. The management of malignant ureteral obstruction treated with ureteral stents. *J. Urol.* 2006;174:2125–8.

Gayed, B. A., Mally, A. D., Riley, J., Ost, M. C. Resonance metallic stents do not effectively relieve extrinsic ureteral compression in pediatric patients. *J. Endourol.* 2013 Feb.;27(2):154-7

Gibbons, R. P., Correa, R. J. Jr, Cummings, K. B., Mason, J. T. Experience with indwelling ureteral stent catheters. *J. Urol.* 1976;115:22-6.

Goldsmith, Z. G., Wang, A. J., Bañez, L. L., Lipkin, M. E., Ferrandino, M. N., Preminger, G. M., Inman, B. A. Outcomes of metallic stents for malignant ureteral obstruction. *J. Urol.* 2012 Sep.;188(3):851-5.

Harding, J. R. Percutaneous antegrade ureteric stent insertion in malignant disease. *Clin. Radiol.* 1995 Jan.;50(1):68

Hendlin, K., Vedula, K., Horn, C., Monga, M. In vitro evaluation of ureteral stent compression. *Urology* 2006 Apr.: 67:679-82

Hendlin, K., Korman, E., Monga, M. New metallic ureteral stents: improved tensile strength and resistance to extrinsic compression. *J. Endourol.* 2012 Mar.;26(3):271-4.

Kim, J. H., Song, K., Jo, M. K., Park, J. W. Palliative care of malignant ureteral obstruction with polytetrafluoroethylene membrane-covered self-expandable metallic stents: initial experience. *Korean J. Urol.* 2012 Sep.; 53(9):625-31.

Klarskov, P., Nordling, J., Nielsen, J. B. Experience with Memokath 051 ureteral stent. *Scand. J. Urol. Nephrol.* 2005;39:169-72.

Li, C. C., Li, J. R., Huang, L. H., et al. Metallic stent in the treatment of ureteral obstruction: experience of single institute. *J. Chin. Med. Assoc.* 2011 Oct.;74(10):460-3.

Liatsikos, E., Kagadis, G., Barbalias, G., Siablis, D. Ureteral metal stents: a tale or a tool? *J. Endourol.* 2005 Oct.: 19:934-9

Liatsikos, E., Kallidonis, P., Kyriazis, I., Constantinidis, C., Hendlin, K., Stolzenburg, J. U., et al. Ureteral obstruction: Is the full metallic double-pigtail stent the way to go? *Eur. Urol.* 2010;57:480-6.

Liatsikos, E. N., Karnabatidis, D., Katsanos, K., Kallidonis, P., Katsakiori, P., Kagadis, G. C., Christeas, N., Papathanassiou, Z., Perimenis, P., Siablis, D. Ureteral metal stents: 10-year experience with malignant ureteral obstruction treatment. *J. Urol.* 2009 Dec.;182(6):2613-7

López-Huertas, H. L., Polcari, A. J., Acosta-Miranda, A., Turk, T. M. Metallic ureteral stents: A cost-effective method of managing benign upper tract obstruction. *J. Endourol.* 2010;24:483-5.

Miyaoka, R., Hendlin, K., Monga, M. Resistance to extrinsic compression and maintenance of intraluminal flow in coil-reinforced stents (Silhouette scaffold device): an in-vitro study. *J. Endourol.* 2010; 24:595-8

Modi, A., Ritch, C., Arend, D., et al. Multicenter experience with metallic ureteral stents for malignant and chronic benign ureteral obstruction. *J. Endourol.* 2010; 24:1189-93

Okeke, Z., Smith, A. D. Malignant ureteral obstruction: the case for plastic ureteral stents. *J. Endourol.* 2008; 22(9):2101-3; discussion 2105-6.

Pauer, W., Lugmayr, H. Metallic Wallstents: A new therapy for extrinsic ureteral obstruction. *J. Urol.* 1992;148:281-4.

Pedro, R. N., Hendlin, K., Kriedberg, C., Monga, M. Wire-based ureteral stents: Impact on tensile strength and compression. *Urology* 2007; 70: 1057–1059.

Polcari, A., Hugen, C., López-Huertas, H., Turk, T. Cost analysis and clinical applicability of the Resonance metallic ureteral stent. *Expert. Rev. Pharmacoecon. Outcomes Res.* 2010 Feb.: 10:11-5

Rao, M. V., Polcari, A. J., Turk, T. M. Updates on the use of ureteral stents: focus on the Resonance® stent. *Med. Devices* (Auckl.). 2011;4:11-5.

Rosenberg, B. H., Bianco, F. J. Jr, Wood, D. P. Jr, Triest, J. A. Stent-change therapy in advanced malignancies with ureteral obstruction. *J. Endourol.* 2005 Jan.-Feb.;19(1):63-7

Sountoulides, P., Kaplan, A., Kaufmann, O. G., Sofikitis, N. Current status of metal stents for managing malignant ureteric obstruction. *BJU Int.* 2010; 105:1066-72

Sountoulides, P., Pardalidis, N., Sofikitis, N. Endourologic management of malignant ureteral obstruction: indications, results, and quality-of-life issues. *J. Endourol.* 2010;24(1):129-42.

Taylor, E. R., Benson, A. D., Schwartz, B. F. Cost analysis of metallic ureteral stents with 12 months of follow-up. *J. Endourol.* 2012 Jul.;26(7):917-21.

Tekin, M. I., Aytekin, C., Aygün, C., PeSkircio~lu, L., Boyvat, F., Ozkarde, H. Covered metallic ureteral stent in the management of malignant ureteral obstruction: preliminary results. *Urology* 2001; 58: 919–23

Trueba Arguinarena, F. J., del Busto, E. F. Self-expanding polytetrafluoroethylene covered nitinol stents for the treatment of ureteral stenosis: preliminary report. *J. Urol.* 2004; 172: 620–3

Wah, T. M., Irving, H. C., Cartledge, J. Initial experience with the resonance metallic stent for antegrade ureteric stenting. *Cardiovasc. Intervent. Radiol.* 2007;30:705–710.

Wilson, J. R., Urwin, G. H., Stower, M. J. The role of percutaneous nephrostomy in malignant ureteric obstruction. *Ann. R Coll. Surg. Engl.* 2005 Jan.;87(1):21-4.

Yachia, D. Recent advances in ureteral stents. *Curr. Opin. Urol.* 2008;18:241–246.

In: Ureters: Anatomy, Physiology and Disorders   ISBN: 978-1-62808-874-8
Editors: R. A. Santucci and M. Chen   © 2013 Nova Science Publishers, Inc.

Chapter 6

Conservative Management of Upper Urinary Tract Transitional Cell Carcinoma

A. Simonato, A. Benelli, M. Ennas and G. Carmignani
Department of Urology, "L. Giuliani", University of Genoa, Italy

Abstract

Upper Urinary Tract Transitional Cell Carcinoma (UUTTCC) is an uncommon disease representing approximately 5% of all urothelial tumors and 1-2% of all genitourinary tumors.

Radical nephroureterectomy is still considered the gold standard treatment for these tumors. However, the radical surgery has been increasingly challenged in the last few years by oncological comparisons with segmental ureterectomy tecniques and endourological treatments. These kidney-sparing surgeries have been used in patients with imperative indications such as solitary kidneys, impaired renal function or synchronous bilateral tumors. Due to the encouraging oncological results, conservative techniques have also been proposed in patients with no imperative indications. Nevertheless, there is a lack of data in the current literature to provide strong recommendations due to the rarity of the disease. Some recent multicenter studies are available but most of these are retrospective. The aim of this review is to assess the efficacy of conservative treatments in reference to oncological outcomes and to elucidate the pertinence of surgical indications.

Introduction

Upper Urinary Tract Transitional Cell Carcinoma (UUT TCC) is an uncommon disease.

It represents less than 1% of genitourinary neoplasms and 5% of all urinary tract tumors with an estimated incidence of 1-4 cases per 100,000 individuals per year. The incidence increases with age in both genders, with a peak diagnosis between the sixth and seventh decades of life [1, 2]. Laterality is approximately equally distributed between right and left sides and about 2-4% of cases are bilateral [3]. Though surgical management of UUT TCC has significantly evolved and improved over the past two decades, radical nephroureterectomy (RNU) with bladder cuff excision has represented the treatment for UUT TCC for more than 60 years, and according to the literature, it is still considered the gold standard treatment [3,4]. The rationale for this treatment is the frequency of multifocality, significant ipsilateral recurrences and relatively low incidence of contralateral involvement [5]. By eliminating the risk of ipsilateral recurrence, radical surgery also requires less frequent follow-up examinations, reducing costs.

Conservative strategies such as segmental ureterectomy (SU) and endourological management have been developed in the last two decades and are now commonly proposed in patients with imperative indications such as solitary kidneys, severely impaired renal function, bilateral synchronous tumors and the future necessity for chemotherapy. Considering the good oncological results achieved for these patients and the fact that a kidney sparing approach could protect from mortality due to other causes, a conservative approach has also been proposed for patients with no imperative indications [6, 7, 8].

In the European Association of Urology Guidelines, the conservative management for UUT TCC with both approaches, open and endoscopic, is accepted only for carefully selected patients.

The topic of standard RNU vs alternative therapy has lost none of its importance or current relevance and it is still considered a matter of debate. Due to the rarity of the disease there are no randomized clinical trials in literature and only a few series reporting long term survival data.

The aim of this chapter is to review the current conservative approaches and oncological outcomes for UUT TCC in efforts to clarify indications for conservative management.

We conducted a Medline search using the National Library of Medicine database using the combination of the following search terms: urothelial carcinoma, transitional cell, upper urinary tract, endoscopic, percutaneous, ureterectomy, kidney sparing surgery, and conservative management; we considered papers between 1990 and 2012, excluding reviews, case reports and papers not written in English. A total of 45 papers were eligible for final evaluation.

Results

We identified a total of 45 articles in the literature, 18 of which discussed segmental resection (Table 1); 27 reviewed the endoscopic approach (Table 2). Both of these approaches are gaining importance in the last two decades due to the association of good oncological results and minimal invasiveness while preserving kidney function. A total of 2054 patients were identified, 1137 of whom underwent segmental ureterectomy. The mean study size for the open approach is 63.2 patients (range 4-569), but only 2 institutions have published series with more than 50 patients with a mean follow-up time longer than 50 months. The endoscopic approach was used in the remaining 917 patients. The mean study size is 34 patients (range 6-90) and only 5 institutions have published series with more than 50 patients with a mean follow-up longer than 50 months.

It is difficult--and in some cases statistically incorrect--to compare the outcomes of all these studies due to their data heterogeneity. For example, follow-up durations are variably expressed as mean or median in the different studies. Furthermore, many of the studies did not use tumor location as a selection criterion or simply did not indicate it in the preoperative data. As a result, survival could not be stratified by tumor location. The most homogenous and significant information we could glean from the collective data was the 5 year cancer specific survival (CsS) rate. Unfortunately, in most cases, CSS was not stratified for stage and grade of the disease.

Another key point regarding the oncological outcome of UUT TCC is the recurrence rate. According to the European Association of Urology Guidelines, RNU is considered the gold standard treatment regardless of the location of the tumor in the upper urinary tract; it eliminates the risk of ipsilateral recurrence and requires a less strict follow-up. The conservative management of UUT TCC can be commonly proposed in imperative cases such as patients with solitary kidney or renal insufficiency. However, these indications are softening due to the encouraging oncological results of segmental ureterectomy.

Table 1. Segmental ureterectomy for UUT TCC in literature

Authors/year	Patients N°	Median/mean f-up (mths)	Stage (N° patients)	5 yrs cancer-spec survival	5 yrs bladder-rec. free survival
Maier et al. (1990) [20]	52	41,4	Ta(15), T1(21), T2(11), T3(4), T4(1)	69,2% (41,4mths)	*
Das et al. (1990) [21]	10	Long term	A(5), B(3), D(2)	*	*
Bukurov et. al (1992) [22]	101[1]	1-14 yrs	*	73%	*
Bouffioux et al. (1994) [23]	20[2]	41	Ta(7), T1(9), T2(2), T3(2)	90%	*
Racioppi et al. (1997) [24]	47	75	*	25% (15yrs)	62%
Hall et al. (1998) [25]	36	64	*	23%	*
Fujimoto et al. (1999) [26]	10	83,5	Tis(1),Ta(1), T1(4), T2(1), T3(2)	91,7%	60% at 83 mths
Chen et al. (2005) [27]	12	49,3[3]	Ta(1), T1(11)	46,4%[3]	66.6%
van der Poel. (2005) [28]	36	81	*	*	*
Roupert et al. (2007) [29]	6	32	Ta(5), T2(1)	100%	83,3% at 46 mths
Raman et al. (2007) [30]	18	44,1[3]	*	*	*
Giannarini et al. (2007) [31]	19	58	Ta(13), T2(4), T3(2)	64%	82%
Lehman et al. (2007) [32]	51	96	Ta(17), T1(14), T2(9), T3(3), T4(5)	80% (10yrs)	*
Dragicevic et al. (2009) [33]	21	67	T1(7), T2(10), T3(4)	55%[3]	*
Eandi et al. (2010) [34]	4	30,5	Tis(1), T1(2), T2(1)	100%	*
Jeldres et al. (2010) [11]	569	30	T1(231), T2(192), T3(124), T4(22)	86,6%	*
Colin et al. (2012) [2]	52	26	Ta(22), T1(12), T2(12), T3(5), T4(1)	87,9%	*
Simonato et al. (2012) [9]	73	87	Ta(31), T1(23), T2(13), T3(26)	94,1%	82.2%

*Data not specified in the article, [1]including partial nephrectomy, [2]including endoscopic approach, [3]including radical approach.

Table 2. Endoscopic conservative treatment for UUT TCC in literature

Authors/year	Approach	Patients N°	Median/mean f-up (mths)	P stage (N° patients)	5 yrs cancer-spec survival
R.M.Moldwin et al. (1990) [35]	Pcn	18	27	*	89% at 27 mths
H.B.Grossmann et al. (1992) [36]	Urs	8	*	*	100%
R.P.Kaufman et al. (1993) [37]	Urs	9	28	9Ta	100%
J.Andresen et al. (1994) [38]	Urs	10	25	*	100%
G. Bales et al. (1994) [39]	4Pcn,2Urs	6	37	*	100%
A. Patel et al. (1996) [40]	Pcn	26	45	5Tx,1Tis,8Ta,10T1,2T2	91% at 3 yrs
D. Elliot et al. (1996) [41]	7Pcn,37Urs	44	52	13Tis,7T1#	73%
F.Keeley et al. (1997) [42]	Urs	38	26	*	*
M.L. Stoller et al. (1997) [43]	4Pcn,16Urs	20	25	*	100% at 25 mths
M. Grasso et al. (1999) [44]	Urs	11	17	*	100% at 17 mths
M.E. Jabbour et al. (2000) [45]	Pcn	59	48	*	95%
M.C. Goel et al. (2003) [46]	Pcn	24	64	*	*
K. Matsuoka et al. (2003) [47]	Urs	20	33	*	95% at 33 mths
S. Daneshmand et al. (2003) [48]	Urs	30	38	*	96,7% at 38 mths
J. Palou et al. (2004) [49]	Pcn	34	51	6T1, 6T1, 22Tx	94,1% at 51 mths
S. Mugiya et al. (2006) [50]	Urs	7	30	*	71% at 30 mths
M. Roupret et al. (2006) [51]	27Urs,16Pcn	43	51	22Ta,3Tis,11T1,6T2,1T3	80%
M. Roupret et al. (2006) [52]	Pcn	24	62	10Ta,2Tis,8T1,3T2,1T3	79.5%
A.E. Krambeck et al. (2007) [53]	Urs	90	51	*	81%
S.J. Sowter et al. (2007) [54]	37Pcn,4Urs	40	42	*	100%
R.H. Thompson et al. (2008) [55]	Pcn,Urs	83	55	78Ta, 3Tis, 2T1	85.4%
R.H. Thompson et al. (2008) [56]	Urs	22	59	22Ta	89.6%
R.W. Pak et al. (2009) [19]	Urs,Pcn	57	53	*	94.7%
A.J. Gadzinski et al. (2010) [57]	Urs,Pcn	34	77	*	100%
E.M. Raymundo et al. (2011) [58]	Urs,Pcn	21	18	16T1,2T2,3T4	95% at 18 mths
M. Grasso et al. (2012) [18]	Urs	66	52	*	87%
M.L. Cutress et al. (2012) [17]	Urs,Pcn	73	54	14Tx,56Ta,3T1	88.9%

*Data not specified in the article.

The current indications include unifocal, small, low grade tumors, with no evidence of infiltrative lesions on computer tomography with close follow-up [3]. Cancer recurrence-free survival is a rare event. It was reported in 5 articles regarding segmental ureterectomy, but only 4 had success expressed as 5 year survival.

Tumor location in the urinary tract plays an important role in the type of treatment. Ureteral tumors can be treated with ureteroscopy. Renal pelvic and calyceal tumors are amenable to open partial resection and percutaneous endoscopic resection.

Discussion

To date, there are no prospective randomized studies in the literature regarding the conservative approach to UUT TCC. Moreover, due to the rarity of the disease, it is not common to find studies enrolling a proper number of patients with good follow-up duration. Also, complete information about the tumor stage and recurrence-free survival is lacking. This results in incomplete data regarding the most appropriate management of the disease.

Open Segmental Resection

Open segmental resection is commonly proposed for ureteral tumors, preferably when the disease involves the distal part of the ureter. Open resection of the renal pelvis or calyxes has all but disappeared [9]. Since the pioneering work of Zincke [10] at the Mayo clinic 30 years ago, growing attention to the encouraging oncological results offered by the conservative approach to these tumors has been observed and different techniques of open segmental ureterectomy have been described and developed over the years. Regarding this approach, it should certainly be emphasized that the segmental resection of the iliac and lumbar ureter is associated with a higher failure rate than that of the distal pelvic ureter.

The approximate location and extension of the tumor are studied with preoperative imaging and ureteroscopy. This information will allow the surgeon to choose the most appropriate technique. The choice of a refluxing or non-refluxing anastomosis is still controversial: the first allows an easier follow-up of the upper urinary tract, while the second may avoid urinary infections and cell spillage from the bladder to the upper urinary tract [3].

The end-to-end anastomosis is the simplest technique and can be used for small tumors involving a short portion of the ureter. Oftentimes, frozen sections are sent intraoperatively in order to avoid positive margins. Direct ureterocystostomy is possible only when a short segment (3-4 cm) of the intramural and juxtavesical ureter is involved. Most of the time, the extravesical technique described by Litch is preferred, reducing the risk of urinary fistula. The bladder psoas muscle hitch can treat tumors involving up to 4-5 cm of the distal ureter. A Boari flap can be used for longer segment ureteral involvement. Should all these techniques prove insufficient, ileal ureteral substitution can be used. The indications for laparoscopic and robotic distal ureterectomy are the same as those for the open approach, and the choice for the laparoscopic approach is mostly dependent on the surgeon's experience.

The aim of this chapter is to clarify doubts about long term oncological outcome in patients with UUT TCC treated with a conservative approach. In a recent study, Jeldres et al. demonstrated a lack of inferiority in terms of cancer specific survival when segmental ureterectomy (SU) is compared to radical nephroureterectomy (RNU) with or without bladder cuff excision. SU was performed in 569 patients while RNU was performed in 1475 (1222 with bladder cuff excision and 253 without). They obtained a CSS at 5 years respectively of 86.6%, 82.2% and 80.5%. In the multivariable Cox regression analyses of CSS, the surgery type failed to reach independent predictor status. They also stratified CSS according to the stage of the disease in patients with pT1-2 and pT3-4 tumors, obtaining a CSS at 5 years for SU of 91.2% and 71.9% respectively. No difference was noted when SU was compared to RNU in the two groups [11]. This paper contains the largest series of SU compared to RNU for UUT TCC, though there are several limitations related to the usage of a population-based tumor registry: 1) there is absence of information about the localization of the tumors in the urinary tract and about recurrence-free survival (RFS); 2) bladder recurrence-free survivals (BRFS) are not reported. The risk of recurrence is a very important issue, strongly related to the importance of an accurate follow-up in patients who undergo a conservative approach for UUT TCC. Simonato et al. obtained a bladder recurrence-free survival at 5 years of 82.2% in a series of 73 patients treated with SU, comparable with data in the literature for RNU [9]. Colin et al. found no statistically significant difference in terms of RFS and metastasis-free survival (MFS) at 5 years between their series of 52 patients treated with SU and 416 treated with RNU. They also performed a subgroup analysis regarding unifocal, small and low clinical stage tumors of the distal ureter with positive surgical margin being the only independent prognostic factor for RFS and MFS [2]. Ku et al. also indicated the prognostic value of positive surgical margins in univariate analyses for CSS [12].

According to the literature good oncological results in terms of CSS could also be obtained in patients with more advanced stage disease (pT3-T4) when treated with segmental ureterectomy. The data suggested that these patients should not be excluded from consideration for conservative surgery and could be potential candidates for this approach [9, 11, 12]. Certainly, these results must be interpreted with caution mainly because of the small number of cases, the likelihood of a selection bias, and potential error in the preoperative clinical staging of these patients.

Endoscopic Approaches

The endoscopic treatment of UUT TCC can be performed via a retrograde ureteroscopic or percutaneous antegrade approach. According to the reported literature, the first conservative treatment of an UUT TCC of the renal pelvis with an endoscopic retrograde approach was performed in 1984 by Goodman. Three years later, Bagley published his innovative work on the study of diagnostic and therapeutic URS [13]. In the same year, the first percutaneous treatment of UUT TCC was proposed [14,15]. Nowadays, it is possible to endoscopically access the entire urinary tract due to technologic advancements in ureteroscopic instruments and surgical techniques. We can now benefit from flexible ureteropyeloscopy, which are available in sizes smaller than 8 Fr. Rigid ureteroscopes are used in the distal and middle ureter since they provide better visualization than the flexible ones due to their larger diameter, which allows greater irrigant flow and the use of larger operative instruments. According to the EAU guidelines, laser ablation of UUT TCC with Nd:YAG or Ho:YAG lasers permit resection of large tumors with good hemostasis [15,16].

Historically, much like for open segmental resection, the indications for endoscopic treatment of UUT TCC are expanding. Once reserved only for a small number of cases due to specific requirements, nowadays endoscopic management has been extended to carefully selected patients with elective indications. These include small, unifocal tumors of low grade and low clinical stage with a contralateral functioning kidney [2, 17]. The choice between ureteroscopy and percutaneous nephroscopy essentially depends on tumor location and size.

Usually, ureteroscopy is preferred for small ureteral and renal pelvic tumors while the anterograde percutaneous approach is better for larger tumors (large pelvic tumors, bulky tumors of the proximal ureter), tumors that cannot be reached through the retrograde route (such as in the lower pole calyxes), and in patients with previous urinary diversion. Nevertheless ureteroscopy is a closed-system approach to the upper urinary tract and offers lower morbidity than the percutaneous route [2, 14, 16].

It should be remembered that there are no known randomized trials comparing endoscopic management with RNU; all published reports are non-randomized studies. According to our search results, the mean study size was 34 patients with only 5 institutions having published series with more than 50 patients with a mean follow-up longer than 50 months. As a result of these observations, the topic of conservative treatment versus RNU still remains relatively unclear as it is hard to draw any definitive conclusions on the long term oncological efficacy of the conservative approach. Cutress et al. demonstrated that the endoscopic approach seems to offer effective long term oncological control with an acceptable CSS of 88.9% at 5 years in well selected patients. This paper also evaluated tumor grade, and not surprisingly, CSS reduced significantly with increasing grade. Also, Gadzinski in his work, showed how CSS and MFS were strongly associated with grade at presentation moreso than with the type of surgery [17].

Grasso presented his work on 82 patients that were divided into 2 groups: the first one included 66 electively treated tumors with a CSS of 87% at 5 years; the second group had 16 patients treated with a palliation goal with a resultant lower CSS of 54% at 2 years [18]. The author compares these two groups with a third group that includes 80 patients treated with RNU that had a CSS of 64% at 5 years. The CSS rates for low grade tumors at 5 years treated with URS and RNU were similar, with an increasing but not significant difference at 10 years [18].

Bladder and ureteral recurrences are a very important issue in the conservative approach to UUT TCC. Cutress obtained a bladder-free recurrence survival of 68.9%, with grading and previous TCC of the bladder being the only independent prognostic factors for BRFS [17]. According to the literature, multivariate analysis has shown the following factors as significant for UT recurrences: grade, multifocality, prior bladder tumors and tumor size.

One of the most discussed aspects of the radical approach compared to the conservative one is the fact that it provides cheaper follow-up costs. Cost analysis of conservative management was reported by Pak. He estimated the average cost of saving a kidney to be 117,890 US dollars over a followup of

53 months, with consideration given to the average recurrence rate at his institution over this time period [19]. Radical surgery was initially cheaper, but the increased need for hemodialysis and fistula creation has a projected 5 year cost estimated at 385,145 US dollars.

UUT TCCs are considered high recurrence rate tumors. In order to reduce recurrence risk after conservative treatment, adjuvant topical instillation therapy with the same agents used for TCC (Mitomycin and BCG) of the bladder can be considered. The goal of this treatment is for continued exposure of the urothelium to the topical agent. The cumulative experience appears encouraging [15,16]. Nevertheless, there is no randomized control trial establishing a standardized regimen.

Conclusion

UUT TCC is a rare tumor with a substantial lack of data in the current literature regarding patients undergoing conservative management. There are only a few retrospective non-randomized studies with a good number of patients and acceptable duration of follow-up; no randomized trials comparing the conservative and radical approach have yet been conducted. It is difficult to compare the outcomes of various retrospective studies, due to the differences in the selection criteria of patients, treatment indications, follow-up duration and data stratification. However, after analysis of the current literature, we believe it is possible to draw several conclusions to clarify doubts about the conservative management of UUT TCC. Before choosing the optimal treatment, urologists should take into account the characteristics of each patient with regard to: tumor stage and grade, localization of the lesion, patients' comorbidities, and renal function. Segmental ureterectomy, when technically feasible, is a good option. It offers good cancer control with 5 years CSS comparable to RNU in patients with single, unifocal, low stage and grade tumor of the distal ureter. For specific cases (low grade and low volume tumors affecting the proximal ureter or the calicopyelic system), endoscopic management seems to provide effective oncologic control and preserve renal function. Unfortunately, the long-term outcomes are currently undefined. Recurrences are common and occur in most patients, making periodic endoscopic follow-up mandatory.

References

[1]   M. Ozsahin, G. Ugurluer, A. Zouhair. Management of transitional-cell carcinoma of the renal pelvis and ureter. *SWISSM EDWKLY* 2009; 139(25–26):353–356.

[2]   P. Colin, A. Ouzzane, G. Pignot et al. Comparison of oncological outcomes after segmental ureterectomy or radical nephroureterectomy in urothelial carcinomas of the upper urinary tract: results from a large French multicentre study. *BJU Int* 2012; 110: 1134–41.

[3]   M. Roupret, M. Babjukb, E. Comperat, R. Zigeuner, R. Sylvester, M. Burger, N. Cowang, A. Bohle, B. W.G. Van Rhijni, E. Kaasinenj, J. Palouk, S. F. Shariatl. European Guidelines on Upper Tract Urothelial Carcinomas: 2013 Update. *European urology Volume 63*, Issue 6, June 2013, 1059–1071.

[4]   M. L. Blute, J. Segura, D. Patterson, R.C. Benson, H. Zincke. Impact of endourology on diagnosis and management of upper urinary tract urothelial cancer. *J. Urol* 1989;141:1298–301.

[5]   Z. Kirkali, E. Tuzel. Transitional cell carcinoma of the ureter and renal pelvis. *Critical Reviews in Oncology/Hematology* 47 (2003) 155,169.

[6]   D. S. Elliott, JW Segura, D Lightner, DE Patterson, ML Blute. Is nephroureterectomy necessary in all cases of upper tract transitional cell carcinoma? Long-term results of conservative endourologic management of upper tract transitional cell carcinoma in individuals with a normal contralateral kidney. Urology 2001; 58:174 – 8.

[7]   I. Iborra, E. Solsona, J. Casanova, J.V. Ricos, J. Rubio, M.A. Climent. Conservative elective treatment of upper urinary tract tumors: a multivariate analysis of prognostic factors for recurrence and progression. *J. Urol* 2003; 169:82 – 5.

[8]   L. Zini, P. Perrotte, U. Capitanio et al: Radical versus partial nephrectomy: effect on overall and non cancer mortality. *Cancer* 2009; 115: 1465.

[9]   A. Simonato ,V. Varca, A. Gregori, A. Benelli, M. Ennas, A. Lissiani, M. Gacci, S. De Stefani, M. Rosso, S. Benvenuto, G. Siena, E. Belgrano, F. Gaboardi, M. Carini, G. Bianchi and G. Carmignani. Elective segmental ureterectomy for transitional cell carcinoma of the ureter: long-term follow up in a series of 73 patients. *BJUITERNATIONAL* 2012. 110, E 744–E 749.

[10] H. Zincke, R.J. Neves. Feasibility of conservative surgery for transitional cell cancer of the upper urinary tract. *Urol. Clin. North Am.* 1984; 11: 717 – 24.

[11] C. Jeldres, G. Lughezzani, Sun M. et al., Segmental ureterectomy can safely be performed in patients with transitional cell carcinoma of the ureter. *J. Urol.* 2010; 183: 1324–9.

[12] J. H. Ku, W.S. Choi, C. Kwak and H.H. Kim: Bladder cancer after nephroureterectomy in patients with urothelial carcinoma of the upper urinary tract. *Urol. oncol.* 2011; 29:383-7.

[13] D. H. Bagley, JL Huffman, ES Lyon.Flexible ureteropyeloscopy: diagnosis and treatment in the upper urinary tract. *J. Urol.* 1987; 138: 280 – 5.

[14] B. T. Ristau, Jeffrey J. Tomaszewski, and M. C. Ost. Upper Tract Urothelial Carcinoma:Current Treatment and Outcomes. *Urology* 79: 749–756, 2012. Elsevier Inc.

[15] G. Cai, X. Liu, B. Wu. Treatment of upper urinary tract urothelial carcinoma. *Surgical Oncology* (2011) 20,43,55.

[16] M. L. Cutress, G. D. Stewart, P. Zakikhani, S. Phipps, B. G. Thomas and D. A. Tolley. Ureteroscopic and percutaneous management of upper tract urothelial carcinoma (UTUC): systematic review. *Bjuinternational* 2012.110,614–628.

[17] M. L. Cutress, G. D. Stewart, S. Wells-Cole, S. Phipps, B. G. Thomas and D. A. Tolley. Long-term endoscopic management of upper tract urothelial carcinoma: 20-year single-centre experience. 2012 *Bjuinternational*, 110,1608–1617.

[18] M. Grasso, M. I. Fishman, J. Cohen and B. Alexander. Ureteroscopic and extirpative treatment of upper urinary tract urothelial carcinoma: a 15-year comprehensive review of 160 consecutive patients. 2012 *Bjuinternational*, 110,1618–1626.

[19] R. W. Pak, E. J. Moskowitz, and D. H. Bagley. What Is the Cost of Maintaining a Kidney in Upper-Tract Transitional-Cell Carcinoma? An Objective Analysis of Cost and Survival. *Journal of Endourology* V. 23, N. 3, March 2009, 341-346.

[20] U. Maier, G. Mertl, K. Pummer. Organ-preserving surgery in patients with urothelial tumors of the upper urinary tract. *Eur. Urol.* 1990; 18:197 – 200.

[21] A. K. Das, C.C. Carson, D. Bolick, D.F. Paulson. Primary carcinoma of the upper urinary tract: effect of primary and secondary therapy on survival. *Cancer* 1990; 66: 1919 – 23.

[22] N. Bukurov, K. Stefanovic, S. Petkovic. Justifiability of conservative surgery for transitional cell carcinoma of the upper urinary tract. *Prog. Clin. Biol. Res.* 1992; 378 : 145 – 52.

[23] C. H. Bouffioux, R. Adrianne, P. Bonnet et al. The experience of the CHU Li é ge with conservative surgery in the management of upper urinary tract tumors. *Acta Urol Belg* 1994; 62: 39–43.

[24] M. Racioppi, A. D.' addessi, A. Alcini, A. Destito, E. Alcini. Clinical review of 100 consecutive surgically treated patients with upper urinary tract. Transitional tumors. *BJU* 1997; 80: 707–11.

[25] M. C. Hall, S. Womack, A.I. Sagalowsky, T. Carmody, M.D. Erickstad, C.G. Roehrborn. Prognostic factors, recurrence, and survival in transitional cell carcinoma of the upper urinary tract: a 30-year experience in 252 patients. *Urology* 1998; 52: 594 – 601.

[26] N. Fujimoto, H. Sato, A. Mizokami, H. Inatomi, T. Matsumoto. Results of conservative treatment of upper urinary tract transitional cell carcinoma. *Int. J. Urol.* 1999; 6: 381 – 7.

[27] W. J. Chen, J.Y. Kuo, K.K. Chen, A.T.L. Lin, Y.H. Chang, L.S. Chang. Primary urothelial carcinoma of the ureter: 11-year experience in Taipei Veterans General Hospital. *J. Chin. Med. Assoc.* 2005; 68: 522 – 30.

[28] H. G. Van der Poel, N. Antonini, H. van S Tinteren, Horenblas. Upper urinary tract cancer: location is correlated with prognosis. *Eur. Urol.* 2005; 4 8: 438 – 44.

[29] M. Rouprêt, J.D. Harmon, K.M. Sanderson et al. Laparoscopic distal ureterectomy and anastomosis for management of low risk upper urinary tract transitional cell carcinoma: preliminary results. *BJU Int* 2007; 99: 623 – 7.

[30] J. D. Raman, R.E. Sosa, E.D. Vaughan, D.S. Scherr. Pathologic features of bladder tumors after nephroureterectomy or segmental ureterectomy for upper urinary tract transitional cell carcinoma. *Urology* 2007; 69:251–4.

[31] G. Giannarini, M.C. Schumacher, G.N. Thalmann, A. Bitton, A. Fleischmann, UE Studer. Elective management of transitional cell carcinoma of the distal ureter: can kidney-sparing surgery be advised? *BJU Int* 2007; 100: 264 – 8.

[32] J. Lehmann, H. Suttmann, I. Kovac et al. Transitional cell carcinoma of the ureter: prognostic factors infl uencing progression and survival. *Eur. Urol.* 2007; 51: 1281 – 8.

[33] D. Dragicevic, M. Djokic, T. Pekmezovic et al. Comparison of open nephroureterectomy and open conservative management of upper urinary tract transitional cell carcinoma. *Urol. Int* 2009; 82: 335 – 40.

[34] J. A. Eandi, R.A. Nelson, T.G. Wilson, D.Y. Josephson. Oncologic outcomes for complete robot-assisted laparoscopic management of upper-tract transitional cell carcinoma. *J. Endourol* 2010; 24: 969 – 75.

[35] R. M. Moldwin, E. Orihuela, A.D. Smith. Conservative management for transitional cell carcinoma of the upper urinary tract. *Clinics in geriatric medicine*. V.6, N.1, 1990, 163-171.

[36] H. B. Grossman, S.L. Schwartz, J.W. Konnak. Ureteroscopic treatment of urothelial carcinoma of the ureter and renal pelvis. *The journal of urology* V.148, 275-277, 1992.

[37] R. P. Kaufman, C.C Carson.Ureteroscopic management of transitional cell carcinoma of the ureter using the Neodymuium: YAG laser. *Laser in surgery and medicine*, 13:625-628.

[38] J. R. Andersen, J.K. Kristensen.Ureteroscopic management of transitional cell tumors. *Scand jurol nephrol* 28:153-157, 1994.

[39] G. Bales, E. S. Lyon, and G. S. Gerber Conservative Management of Transitional Cell Carcinoma of the Kidney and Ureter. Diagnostic and *Therapeutic Endoscopy*, 1995, Vol. 1, pp. 121-123.

[40] A. Patel, P. Soonawalla, S. F. Shepherd, D. P. Dearnaley, M. J. Kellett and C. R. J. Woodhouse Long-term outcome after percutaneous treatment of transitional cell carcinoma of the renal pelvis. *The Journal of Urology,* Vol. 155,868-874, March 1996.

[41] D. s. Elliott, m. l. Blute, d. e. Patterson, e. j. Bergstralh, and j. w. Segura. Long-term follow-up of endoscopically treated upper urinary tract transitional cell carcinoma. *Urology*, 47-6 1996.

[42] F. Keeley, M. Bibbo and D. h. Bagley. Ureteroscopic treatment and surveillance of upper urinary tfuct transitional cell carcinoma. *The Journal of Urology*. Vol. 157, 1560-1565, May 1997.

[43] Stoller ML, Gentle DL, McDonald MW, Reese JH, Tacker JR, Carroll PR, Best C. Endoscopic management of upper tract urothelial tumors. *Tech Urol.* 1997 Fall;3(3):152-7.

[44] M. Grasso, M. Fraiman, and M Levine Ureteropyeloscopic diagnosis and treatment of upper urinary tract urothelial malignancies., *Urology,* 54 (2), 1999.

[45] M. E. Jabbour, F. Desgrandchamps, S. Cazin, P. Teillac, A. le Duc and A. D. Smith Percutaneous management of grade ii upper urinary tract

transitional cell carcinoma: the long-term outcome. *The Journal of Urology*, Vol. 163, 1105–1107, April 2000.

[46] M. C. Goel, v. Mahendra and J. G. Roberts. Percutaneous management of renal pelvic urothelial tumors: long-term followup. *The Journal of Urology*, Vol. 169, 925–930, March 2003.

[47] K. Matsuoka, S. Lida, K. Tomiyasu, M. Inoue, and S. Noda. Transurethral Endoscopic Treatment of Upper Urinary Tract Tumors Using a Holmium:YAG Laser. *Lasers in Surgery and Medicine* 32:336–340 (2003).

[48] S. Daneshmand, M. L. Quek, J. L. Huffman Endoscopic Management of Upper Urinary Tract Transitional Cell Carcinoma. *Cancer* July 1, 2003 / Volume 98 / Number 1.

[49] J. Palou, L. F. Piovesan, J. Huguet, J. Salvador, J. Vicente and H. Villavicencio Percutaneous nephroscopic management of upper urinary tract transitional cell carcinoma: recurrence and long term followup. *The journal of urology*, vol. 172, 66–69, july 2004.

[50] S. Boorjian, Casey ng, R. Munver, M. A. Palese, E. D. Aughan, R. E. Sosa, J. del Pizzo, and D. Scherr. Impact of delay to nephroureterectomy for patients undergoing ureteroscopic biopsy and laser tumor ablation of upper tract transitional cell carcinoma. *Urology* 66: 283–287, 2005.

[51] M. Rouprêt, V. Hupertan, O. Traxer, G. Loison, E. Chartier-Kastler, P Conort, MC. Bitker, B Gattegno, F. Richard, and O. Cussenot. Comparison of open nephroureterectomy and ureteroscopic and percutaneous management of upper urinary tract transitional cell carcinoma. *Urology* 67 (6), 2006.

[52] M. Roupret, O. Traxer, M. Tligui, P. Conort, E. Chartier-Kastler, F. Richard, O. Cussenot. Upper Urinary Tract Transitional Cell Carcinoma: Recurrence Rate after Percutaneous Endoscopic Resection european urology 51 (2 0 0 7) 709–714.

[53] A. E. Krambeck, Thompson R.H., Lohse C.M., Patterson D.E., Elliott D.S., Blute M.L. Imperative indications for conservative management of upper tract transitional cell carcinoma. *The Journal of Urology.* Volume 178, Issue 3, Pages 792-797, September 2007.

[54] S. J. Sowter, C. P. Ilie, I. Efthimiou, and D. A. Tolley. Endourologic management of patients with upper-tract transitional-cell carcinoma: long-term follow-up in a single center. *Journal of Endourology*, Volume 21, Number 9, September 2007.

[55] R. H. Thompson, A. E. Krambeck, C. M. Lohse, D. S. Elliott, D. E. Patterson, and M. L. Blute. Endoscopic Management of Upper Tract

Transitional Cell Carcinoma in Patients with Normal Contralateral Kidneys. *Urology* 71 (4), 2008.

[56] R. H. Thompson, A. E. Krambeck, C. M. Lohse, D. S. Elliott, D. E. Patterson and M. L. Blute. Elective endoscopic management of transitional cell carcinoma first diagnosed in the upper urinary tract 2008 *BJU International* |102, 1107–1110.

[57] A. J. Gadzinski, W. W. Roberts, G. J. Faerber and J. S. Wolf. Long-Term Outcomes of Nephroureterectomy versus Endoscopic Management for Upper Tract Urothelial Carcinoma. *The Journal of Urology*. Vol. 183, 2148-2153, June 2010.

[58] E. M. Raymundo, M. E. Lipkin, L. B. Banez, J. G. Mancini, D. E. Zilberman, G. M. Preminger and B. A. Inman. The Role of Endoscopic Nephron-Sparing Surgery in the Management of Upper Tract Urothelial Carcinoma. *Journal of Endourology* Volume 25, Number 3, March 2011. P. 377-384.

In: Ureters: Anatomy, Physiology and Disorders   ISBN: 978-1-62808-874-8
Editors: R. A. Santucci and M. Chen   © 2013 Nova Science Publishers, Inc.

Chapter 7

Upper Urinary Tract Dilation in the Neurogenic Bladder

Limin Liao and *Fan Zhang*

Department of Urology, China Rehabilitation Research Center,
Rehabilitation College of Capital Medical University, Beijing, China

Abstract

Urinary incontinence (UI) and vesicoureteral reflux (VUR) are devastating problems for patients with neurogenic bladder dysfunction (NBD) since they often indicate the presence of high bladder pressure. Elevated intravesical pressures can be transmitted to the upper urinary tract (UUT), causing hydronephrosis (HN) and ureteral dilation.

The gold-standard therapy for a small volume, high pressure bladder is bladder augmentation via enterocystoplasty [1]. Although this procedure increases bladder capacity and compliance, it has a high complication rate and requires careful patient selection and effective evaluation of renal function to maximize outcomes [2 3].

The international reflux study group classification is broadly used for grading VUR. However, there is little agreement on the degree of UUT

---

* Correspondence to: Limin Liao, MD, PhD, Address: Department of Urology, China
  Rehabilitation Research Center, 10 Jiaomen Beilu, Fentai District, Beijing, China 100068.
  Tel: +86 10 87569043. Fax: +86 10 67570492. E-Mail: lmliao@263.net.

dilation that signifies HN. The Society for Fetal Urology (SFU) grading system for hydronephrosis, introduced in 1993, is a subjective, 5-point numerical grading system that assigns a grade of 0 to 4 based on the appearance of the calyces, renal pelvis, and renal parenchymal thickness [4]. However, the classification of UUT dilation for NBD is still under discussion. In this chapter, we describe a new UUT dilation classification system and report the outcome of augmentation enterocystoplasty (AE) in 86 NBD patients by using this classification system. As a secondary goal, we hope to standardize methods of grading UUT dilation and HN for NBD.

Keywords: Classification, upper urinary dilation, augmentation enterocystoplasty, neurogenic bladder dysfunction, urodynamics

New Classification of UUT Dilation

We completed a retrospective review of 86 patients (69 males and 17 females, with mean age 27.2 years) who underwent AE in our center between 2005 and 2012. NBD resulted from traumatic spinal cord injury (SCI) in 26 patients, spina bifida (SB) in 48 patients, and other problems (i.e. tumor) in 12 patients. The majority of patients had a long history of illness (more than 10 years). Thirty-seven patients had urodynamically-proven detrusor hyperactivity, 29 showed maximum intravesical pressures above 40 cm H_2O, and 49 had dyssynergia (26 demonstrated VUR at low intravesical pressures less than 10 cm H_2O) with incontinence. A total of 54 patients demonstrated VUR (bilaterally in 25, left in 15 and right in 14) on fluoroscopy. VUR was graded according to the international reflux study group classification (I-II: 17, III-V: 37).

UUT deterioration was a major determinant for AE. Eighty-four patients showed preoperative UUT deterioration, usually manifested by bilateral hydronephrosis. Preoperative HN was defined as dilation of the ureter and renal pelvis with or without secondary changes in the renal parenchyma. Diagnosis of HN requires radiological methods (ultrasound, isotope renography, computed tomography (CT), magnetic resonance imaging (MRI)). All images were reviewed by an uroradiologist. The severity of preoperative HN and ureteral dilation was classified via prior reported methods [5].

We developed a new classification of UUT dilation (Liao's classification):

- Patients with mild dilatation of the renal pelvis and calyces without ureteral dilation were classified as degree 1 (16 cases);
- patients with moderate dilatation of the renal pelvis and calyces and mild ureter dilation were degree 2 (25 cases);
- patients with moderate dilatation of renal pelvis, calyces, and ureter with ureteral tortuosity were degree 3 (24 cases);
- patients with severe dilatation of the renal pelvis and calyces (no maintained papillary impression) and severe ureteric dilation and tortuosity were degree 4 (19 cases).

Cases were then divided into low- and high-grade HN groups. The low-grade HN group included patients with degree 1 or 2, and the high-grade HN group included those with degree 3 or 4.

The UUT functions were assessed using biochemical tests (serum creatinine level). Thirty patients had chronic renal failure, defined as serum creatinine > 1.5 mg/dl (1mg/dl = 88.41umol/l).

Assessments of Liao's Classification of UUT Dilation

We performed augmentation enterocystoplasty (AE) in patients with neurogenic bladder dysfunction (NBD) and analyzed Liao's classification of upper urinary tract (UUT) dilation in these patients.

Surgical Indications

AE was performed alone or in conjunction with ureteral reimplantation (URI). Indications were assessed individually as described in previous literature [6]. Briefly, indications for AE were medically refractory: 1) UUT deterioration due to high bladder storage pressure (> 40 cm H_2O); 2) urinary incontinence (UI) due to small capacity; 3) overactive bladders with or without decreased compliance (< 10 ml/cm H_2O); and 4) VUR. Of these indications, the most important ones were VUR and UI. Indications for URI were VUR grade III or greater in at least one ureter or ureterovesical junction stenosis

(UVJS). If there was UVJS and UUT deterioration in the contralateral ureter on imaging, bilateral URI was performed. URI was also performed when a lower grade VUR was present at low bladder pressures. Ureters were reimplanted into the native bladder. Our preference was to actively perform URI if VUR was present to prevent future renal dysfunction.

Surgical Technique

Methods of bladder augmentation included a "clam-shell" sigmoid (79 cases) or ileal (5 cases) cystoplasty. In addition, 82 patients underwent a concomitant anti-reflux procedure with construction of a hemi-Kock afferent nipple valve in the native bladder.

The native bladder was opened longitudinally and transversely in the coronal plane. An incision was made laterally between the main branches of the inferior vesical vessels anterior to the trigone and ureteric orifice to a point approximately 2 cm from the internal urethral meatus. The anti-reflux operation was performed by intravesical mobilization of the terminal ureter with subsequent reimplantation through a new hiatus and submucosal tunnel. A 20-30 cm long segment of sigmoid colon was isolated with its vascular pedicle, and opened on its antimesenteric border to form a patch. Mucous and stool was removed by irrigation of the sigmoid colon with anhydrous alcohol for 3-5 minutes. The antimesenteric border was incised longitudinally and a detubulized sigmoid patch was created. The detubulized sigmoid patch was then sutured onto the opened bladder with continuous absorbable braided suture in one layer. Stents were placed into each reimplanted ureter. The augmented bladder was decompressed with a urethral catheter.

Postoperatively, we periodically irrigated the augmented bladder with normal saline, which was commenced on the second day via the indwelling catheter to prevent obstruction. Ureteral stents were removed just before a video-urodynamics assessment at 4 weeks. Patients were advised to continue with bladder irrigations regularly even after discharge from hospital using CSIC.

Assessment

Complications and other patient-perceived problems were documented by a postal questionnaire or telephone interview. These included questions regarding continence, need for subsequent urological interventions, medication usage, catheterization habits, bowel function and patient satisfaction. All patients had a serum creatinine test, renal ultrasound and video-urodynamic assessment routinely at 6, 12 and 24 months following the procedure, and annually thereafter. The urodynamic evaluation consisted of simultaneous measurements of intravesical, intra-abdominal, and detrusor pressures, as well as perineal electromyography with patch electrodes, cystography and voiding cystourethrogram according to International Continence Society recommendations. Maximum bladder capacity (MBC) was defined as a strong desire to void, uncomfortable fullness, or incontinence due to involuntary detrusor contraction or low bladder compliance (BC). Maximum detrusor pressure (MDP) was defined as the maximal value of detrusor pressure recorded during each cystometrogram.

When patients started CISC, the frequency of CISC and catheterized volume were recorded. The number of incontinence episodes and pads used per day were assessed. A 6-point Likert scale was used to assess the patients' perspectives of improvement in bladder symptoms. Patients rated their symptoms with choices like "my bladder condition does not cause me any problems at all" and "my bladder condition causes me very severe problems" on a scale of 0 to 5: 0, no problems; 1, very minor problems; 2, minor problems; 3, moderate problems; 4, severe problems; and 5, many severe problems. Improvement was defined as a score decrease of ≥ 1 point.

Liao's classification was used before and after AE surgery, and UUT dilation was compared for each patient before and after AE surgery.

Statistical Analysis

Results were reported as the mean ± standard deviation (SD). Statistical analysis was performed using SPSS 11.5.0 (SPSS, Chicago, IL, USA; 2002) and student's t-test was used to compare the cystometric parameters before and after the operation. Analysis of variance was used to examine patient reported outcomes according to bladder symptoms. Statistical significance was set at $p < 0.05$.

Results

Seventy-seven patients completed the entire 24-month follow-up, while nine patients completed 12-month follow-up. Patients had significant increases in MBC ($p < 0.001$) and BC ($p < 0.001$) and decrease in MDP ($p < 0.001$) (Table 1) compared to pre-operation findings. There was evidence of preoperative chronic renal failure in 30 patients. Paired data showed 27 patients had improvement in UUT function. For those patients with normal UUT function, there was either improvement or stabilization of UUT function, which was seen by following their serum creatinine (Figure 1).

Table 1. Comparison of pre- and post-operative urodynamics in 86 patients who underwent AE

	MBC (ml)	MDP (cm.H2O)	MUPP (cm.H2O)	BC (ml/cm.H2O)
Pre-operation	167.0 ± 137.3	30.4 ± 24.4	82.8 ± 28.9	11.0 ± 17.8
Post-operation				
6 months	354.3 ± 117.8*	20.4 ± 14.4#	67.3 ± 27.8!	35.4± 53.9&
12 months	439.0 ± 100.9*	13.3 ± 9.6#	80.2 ± 26.0	57.1 ± 80.6&
24 months	468.5 ± 60.6*	10.9 ± 4.5#	73.6 ± 22.7	50.9 ± 23.9&

Data were expressed as mean ± SD. Compared to pre-operation, there were significant increases in maximum bladder capacity (MBC) (*$p < 0.001$) and in bladder compliance (BC) (&$p < 0.001$), and significant decreases in the maximum detrusor pressure (MDP) (#$p < 0.05$). There was significant decrease in the maximum urethral pressure profile (MUPP) (!< 0.01) at 6 months postoperatively.

Liao's classification assessment showed improvement in UUT dilation with high-grades (degree 3 or 4) reducing to 17.4% at 24-month follow-up, compared to 51.2% of preoperatively. Of those 30 patients with renal failure, 16 patients with degree 3 or 4 UUT dilation (high-grades) became degree 1 or 2; 8 patients with degree 2 UUT dilation (low-grades) became degree 1 at 24-month follow-up.

All patients took medications such as anticholinergics (tolterodine 2-4 mg twice per day) and antibiotics the first few months. Medications were continued when needed. Patients were treated with CSIC at a frequency of 4.0 ± 0.8 times per day, with mean drainage volumes of 438.7 ± 82.6 ml. Daily incontinence episodes decreased from 4.4 ± 1.4 to 2.6 ± 1.0 ($p < 0.01$) at 24-month follow-up. The number of pads used per day also decreased (Table 2). Bladder symptom scores improved significantly at 6, 12 and 24 months postoperatively.

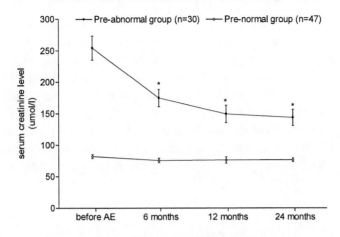

Time chart

The SCL in abnormal group (n = 30) was decreased post-operatively, significant at 6, 12 and 24 months (*p < 0.01). The SCL in normal group (n = 47) was stable postoperatively.

Figure 1. The chronologic change of serum creatinine level (SCL) in patients underwent AE.

Table 2. Comparison of pre- and post-operative urinary incontinence (UI) in 47 patients who underwent sigmoidocolocystoplasty

Category	Pre-operation	Post-operation		
		6 months	12 months	24 months
CSIC				
Frequency (t.p.d)	5.0 ± 1.7	4.8 ± 0.8	3.5 ± 0.7&	4.0 ± 0.8&
Volume each time (ml)	182.4 ± 48.2	386.9 ± 113.9!	454.9 ±106.1!	438.7 ± 82.6!
UI				
Episodes (per day)	4.4 ± 1.4	4.0 ± 1.2	2.5 ± 1.2#	2.6 ± 1.0#
Pads (pieces per day)	4.3 ± 0.6	4.1 ± 0.6	3.0 ± 0.4*	4.2 ± 0.5

Data were expressed as mean ± SD. The clean self-intermittent catheterization (CISC) frequency (times per day, t.p.d) were significantly decreased (&p < 0.05) and catheterized volume each time were significantly increased (!p < 0.01) in post-operation when compared to pre-operation. Compared to the pre-operation, there were significant decreases (#p < 0.01, *p < 0.01) in UI episodes and pads used per day at 12 months.

Complications were classified according to the Clavien scale [7]. Five patients (5.8%) developed adhesive bowel obstruction (Grade 3) distal to or remote from the sigmoid anastamosis. Of those patients with adhesive bowel obstruction, 3 required laparotomy for enterolysis (one required partial resection of the small bowel); one resolved with conservative management; one bowel obstruction was caused by an obstructing band unrelated to the primary procedure. Deterioration in renal function (Grade 4) occurred in three patients (2/3 with preoperative azotemia, 1/3 with poor adherence to a CISC regimen). Persistence of VUR (Grade 2) occurred in 2 patients at 6-month follow-up.

Discussion

The present chapter showed that AE with concomitant URI decreased MDP, increased MBC and BC, and prevented deterioration of UUT with satisfactory patient-reported outcomes during a 24-month follow-up, suggesting that AE has good outcomes in treating patients with NBD.

HN is most commonly classified as mild (5.0 to 9.9 mm), moderate (10.0 to 14.9 mm), or severe ($\geq$15.0 mm) by renal ultrasound. A system to grade HN imaged by ultrasound has been developed and is being used by SFU members in 36 institutions [8]. The appearance of the calyces, renal pelvis and renal parenchyma are key in determining the grade of HN. The present chapter classified UUT dilation into 4 degrees via a new grading system—Liao's classification [5]. Forty-three cases with moderate and severe UUT deteriorations and 27 cases with chronic renal failure demonstrated long-term continued post-operative improvement. Current results indicate that Liao's classification of HN and ureteral dilation is effective in assessing the outcome of AE. It means that Liao's classification can effectively assess the changes of UUT dilation.

It is broadly accepted that significant renal impairment is a more controversial relative contraindication of AE [2, 9]. A recent report suggested AE did not hasten the progression of renal insufficiency in NBD patients [10]. In this chapter, chronic renal failure was found in 3 patients at 24-month follow-up. One patient with preoperative azotemia experienced postoperative renal failure; the patient required dialysis thereafter. It is difficult to discern the etiology of this undesired outcome and it appears to depend on the renal function prior to operation [11]. Skinner et al. recommended that orthotropic urinary diversion should not be offered to patients with significant abnormality in renal function, with a serum creatinine level > 2 mg/dl or creatinine clearance rate < 50 ml/min, to avoid rapid deterioration of renal function after surgery [12]. Long-term indwelling catheterization can be an alternative management strategy [13]. We prefer indwelling transurethral catheters in patients with chronic renal failure (defined as serum creatinine > 1.5 mg/dl) as part of the preoperative preparation and evaluation. If the serum creatinine level gradually decreases, it is more likely to indicate the recovery of renal function postoperatively. This pre-operative evaluation provides patients with severe UUT deterioration a better chance for surgical intervention that may improve renal function.

Neurogenic and non-neurogenic bladders are of different entities. The morphology and innervation of the ureterovesical junction, which play important roles in the incidence of VUR, are different, especially in patients with a long disease history [14]. Long duration NGD and irregular bladder management may account for the high percentage of VUR and UUT deterioration. Decreased compliance secondary to progressive destruction of the bladder wall is an important factor in the etiology of VUR. The majority of our patients had moderate to severe hydronephrosis and/or UUT deterioration at their initial evaluation. In these patients, the short submucosal ureteric tunnel was usually compromised and the UUT function was often not well preserved. Therefore, preoperative evaluation of renal function and HN are important for the management of lower urinary tract disorders. AE alone may not be sufficient to resolve pre-existing VUR. We prefer concomitant URI with AE when significant reflux is present. We also advise early evaluation and management for NBD patients.

Patient-centered outcomes are particularly important following AE, especially since the procedure affects quality of life, especially with changes in continence status. In the present chapter, patient-reported incontinence episodes were related to their bladder symptom scores. The most common problem within 6 months after the operation was incontinence, which may be due to postoperative sphincter weakening. A long-term indwelling urethral catheter could contribute to sphincter weakness as evidenced by a decrease in resting maximum urethral pressure at 6-month follow-up (Table 1). Spontaneous ileal segment contractions of the augmented bladder may also lead to incontinence. Patient perspective outcomes improved after 12 and 24 months, likely because of a decrease in the number of incontinence episodes and pads used per day. Another explanation is that patients may have adapted to their postoperative condition.

During the initial 6-month follow-up, we encountered two patients with persistent or recurrent VUR after reimplantation of the refluxing ureter. The recurrent VUR was successfully cured by anticholinergic therapy with no VUR seen at followup of12- and 24-months. Our experience showed that post-operative VUR is usually caused by UTI and/or increased intravesical pressure. The reimplanted vesical-ureteral junction is vulnerable with risk of ureteric obstruction. Prevention and prompt intervention for UTI should be mandatory. Significant UUT obstruction should be treated by effective urinary drainage. Urine analysis and video-urodynamics assessment are highly recommended at regular intervals, especially in the early phase after surgery.

Most patients with NBD may also have some degree of bowel dysfunction. However, sigmoid cystoplasty appears to have less effect upon bowel function than ileocystoplasty, with dysfunction reported afterward in 6.3% of sigmoid augmentation cystoplasties compared to 55% of ileocystoplasties [15]. Sigmoid augmentation also trended towards lower rates of obstruction when compared with ileum [16]. In the present chapter, five patients (5.8%) presented with adhesive bowel obstruction distal to or remote from the sigmoid anastamosis. Seven patients experienced mild changes of routine bowel programs postoperatively, including increased bowel frequency and looser consistency. Diarrhea or loose stool may happen due to the loss of the terminal part of the colon, causing decreased holding function and fat malabsorption with resultant colonic irritation.

Conclusion

The new classification of UUT dilation (Liao's classification) is effective in assessing the UUT structure and function and the changes in NBD patients. The present chapter indicates that AE is safe for NBD patients with moderate and severe UUT deteriorations. AE may also improve renal function.

Acknowledgments

This chapter was supported in part by grants from the China National Key Technology R&D Program (No.2012BAI34B02) and National Natural Scientific Foundation of China (81070607, 81270847).

References

[1]   Biers SM, Venn SN, Greenwell TJ. The past, present and future of augmentation cystoplasty. *BJU Int.* 2012;109:1280-1293.

[2]   DeFoor W, Minevich E, McEnery P, et al. Lower urinary tract reconstruction is safe and effective in children with end stage renal disease. *J. Urol.* 2003;170: 1497-1500.

[3]   Zhang F, Liao L. Sigmoidocolocystoplasty with ureteral reimplantation for treatment of neurogenic bladder. *Urology.* 2012;80:440-445

[4]   Fernbach SK, Maizels M, Conway JJ. Ultrasound grading of hydronephrosis: introduction to the system used by the Society for Fetal Urology. *Pediatr Radiol.* 1993;23:478-480.

[5]   Liao LM. A Plea for Classification of Comprehensive Urinary Tract Dysfunction for Neurogenic Bladder. *Chinese Journal of Rehabilitation Theory and Practice*, 2010, 16; 1101-1102.

[6]   Hayashi Y, Yamataka A, Kaneyama K, et al. Review of 86 patients with myelodysplasia and neurogenic bladder who underwent sigmoidocolocystoplasty and were followed more than 10 years. *J. Urol.* 2006; 176(4 Pt 2): 1806-1809.

[7]   Dindo D, Demartines N, Clavien PA. Classification of surgical complications: a new proposal with evaluation in a cohort of 6336 patients and results of a survey. *Ann. Surg.* 2004; 240: 205–213.

[8]   Keays MA, Guerra LA, Mihill J, et al. Reliability assessment of society for fetal urology ultrasound grading system for hydronephrosis. *J. Urol.* 2008; 180: 1680-1683.

[9]   Alfrey EJ, Salvatierra O Jr, Tanney DC, et al. Bladder augmentation can be problematic with renal failure and transplantation. *Pediatr. Nephrol.* 1997;11:672-675.

[10] Ivancić V, Defoor W, Jackson E, et al. Progression of renal insufficiency in children and adolescents with neuropathic bladder is not accelerated by lower urinary tract reconstruction. *J. Urol.* 2010;184(4 Suppl):1768-1774.

[11] Greenwell TJ, Venn SN, Mundy AR. Augmentation cystoplasty. *BJU Int.* 2001; 88(6): 511-525.

[12] Skinner DG, Studer UE, Okada K, et al. Which patients are suitable for continent diversion or bladder substitution following cystectomy or other definite local treatment? *Int. J. Urol.* 1995; 2(Suppl 2): 105-112.

[13] Chen JL, Kuo HC. Long-term outcomes of augmentation enterocystoplasty with an ileal segment in patients with spinal cord injury. *J. Formos Med. Assoc.* 2009; 108: 475-480.

[14] Juhasz Z, Somogyi R, Vajda P, et al. Does the Type of Bladder Augmentation Influence the Resolution of Pre-Existing Vesicoureteral Reflux? Urodynamic Studies. *Neurourol. Urodyn.* 2008; 27: 412-416.

[15] N'Dow J, Leung HY, Marshall C, et al. Bowel dysfunction after bladder reconstruction. *J. Urol.* 1998; 159: 1470-1474.

[16] Shekarriz B, Upadhyay J, Demirbilek S, et al. Surgical complications of bladder augmentation: comparison between various enterocystoplasties in 133 patients. *Urology.* 2000;55:123-128.

In: Ureters: Anatomy, Physiology and Disorders   ISBN: 978-1-62808-874-8
Editors: R. A. Santucci and M. Chen   © 2013 Nova Science Publishers, Inc.

Chapter 8

Ureteral Substitution: Evolution from Autologous to Tissue-Engineered Grafts

Matthias D. Hofer[1] and Arun K. Sharma[1-3]*
[1]Northwestern University Feinberg School of Medicine,
Department of Urology, Chicago IL, US
[2]Ann & Robert H. Lurie Children's Hospital of Chicago,
Division of Pediatric Urology, Chicago IL, US
[3]Institute for BioNanotechnology in Medicine (IBNAM),
Chicago IL, US

Abstract

Whereas small defects of the ureter can be addressed by primary repair, more extensive damage requires surgical reconstruction. Procedures such as transuretero-ureterostomy, psoas hitch and Boari flap procedures can be performed for less extensive ureteral damage. Severe injuries with long segment ureteral involvement will require ureteral substitution with ileum or renal autotransplantation. Due to the morbidity of such procedures, synthetic or tissue-engineered grafts have been entertained, used, and continue to be researched. Early results have been disappointing for synthetic grafts prompting exploration of biologic

* E-mail: arun-sharma@northwestern.edu.

scaffolds with stem cell seeding. Yet even these advanced grafts struggle with ensuring appropriate vascular in-growth that is necessary to support the seeded cells long-term and ensure integrity of the tube. Current advances are targeting this problem by using stem cells that have multipotent abilities in differentiation. These cells secrete various growth factors that can stimulate angiogenesis throughout the graft to minimize graft failure. The future for ureteral substitution will therefore be synthetic scaffold membranes seeded with multipotent stem cells that mimic the properties of a normal ureter. These strategies have the potential to obviate the need for ileal ureter substitution and renal autotransplantation. In the following chapter, we review grafts and grafting techniques for ureteral reconstruction with a focus on the current status of tissue-engineered grafts for ureteral reconstruction.

Introduction

Reconstruction of the ureter is necessary for severe ureteral injuries that lead to retroperitoneal urine accumulation with resultant urinoma, abscess, and sepsis. Ureteric obstruction may also occur and result in progressive renal deterioration. Non-iatrogenic ureteral injuries, both blunt and penetrating, have increased in frequency in the past 20 years, partly due to improved patient survival and imaging techniques [1]. Similarly, iatrogenic ureteral injuries, which now comprise about 70% of all ureter injuries, have also been increasing [2]. This is attributed to rising utilization of laparoscopy and ureteroscopy [3]. Most ureteral injuries can be treated with standard techniques such as ureteral stenting, primary anastomosis, vesicopsoas hitch, and Boari bladder flap. More extensive injuries will require renal autotransplantation or ureteral substitution with an ileal segment. Congential anomalies like ureteropelvic junction obstruction and megaureter can often be repaired without substitution.

Ureter obstruction caused by retroperitoneal disease processes such as retroperitoneal fibrosis (RPF) may require ureteral substitution if ureterolysis with or without additional medical management (such as steroids) fails. In addition, RPF associated with vascular aneurysms may prohibit ureterolysis due to an unacceptably high risk of vascular injury. In these cases, ureteral substitution is often necessary. The following chapter describes techniques that utilize grafts for ureteral reconstruction.

Substitution of the Ureter with Autologous Grafts

In the beginning of the 20th century, Strauss described his approach to reconstruct the ureter using a tubularized fragment of transversalis fascia, transversalis muscle, and peritoneum (published in *"Transaction of the section on obstetrics, gynecology and abdominal surgery"* in 1914) [5]. With increasing experience, ileum, colon, and appendix became popular graft tissue for ureter reconstruction. Ureter substituted with ileum remains the best described entity of ureteral substitution, though rare reports of colonic and appendiceal substitution do exist, especially in the pediatric population [6-8].

The first description of the ileal ureter was by Rack in 1953 [9]. Over the following decades, Goodwin et al published their results with success rates as high as 82% when success was defined as stable or decreased serum creatinine or hydronephrosis [10]. Historically, the most common indications for ileal ureter were ureteral damage (22%), intractable urolithiasis (16.5%), bilhariasis (15.5%), radiation fibrosis (8.8%) and gynecological surgery (8.5%) [11]. Current indications are iatrogenic injury due to urologic surgery (31.9%), radiation fibrosis (18.7%), retroperitoneal fibrosis (12.1%), vascular surgery (8.8%), and therapy of urothelial carcinoma (5.5%) [11]. The rising number of repairs for radiation damage of the ureter over the past two decades suggests that this trend will continue. An ileal segment is ideal in this situation due to its uncompromised and reliable blood supply. Current reports describe success rates of 75-100% (combined 177 patients with a mean follow-up of 1.5-3 years) [11-13]. The most common short-term complications included ileus (in up to 15%), urinary tract infection (in up to 14%) and pyelonephritis (25%) [11, 12]. Long-term complications were overall rare and reported as chronic renal failure (reported as 18% by Chung et al. although these patients appeared to have pre-existing azotemia[12]), incisional hernia in 4%-12.5%, fistula formation in 7%, and small bowel obstruction in 4% [11, 12]. Anastomotic strictures were rare (3-6.3%), and development of hyperchloremic metabolic acidosis, reported only by Armatys et al., was seen in 3% of their patients [11, 12]. No patient complained of excessive urinary mucous production. Despite these results, there has been and there always will be hesitation to employ ileal ureters in a widespread manner mainly because of its unfamiliarity to many urologists and the associated risks of gastrointestinal related complications. Another adverse event that may occur is progressive renal deterioration due to recurrent infections, urinary stasis, as well as pressure transduction from bladder outlet obstruction. For example, men with benign prostatic hyperplasia (BPH) should not be treated with ureteral substitution until after their BPH is addressed appropriately. Therefore, this procedure should be limited to patients with normal renal function, pre-operative drainage of an obstructed system, and no evidence of bladder outlet obstruction [13].

Due to the invasiveness and inherent risks of ileal ureter substitution, the search for other suitable ureteral substitution material has been undertaken for over 60 years. Initially, various rigid synthetic materials were used that, over time, were replaced by flexible materials. Further advancements led to engineered structures that increasingly resembled a human ureter.

Development of Synthetic and Semi-Synthetic Grafts

In 1947, Lubash et al. reported on the use of tantalum—a metal with high corrosion resistant properties—for ureteral replacement with poor results [14]. Ulm et al. used Teflon, but these prostheses needed to be explanted in two-thirds of the patients due to severe urinary tract infection or incrustation of the material [15]. Hodge also used Teflon and was able to keep a patent ureter for 5 months [16]. In 1972, Wagenknecht and Auvert implanted Dakron-silicone ureteral prostheses and achieved survival times of more than 4 months, although none of these materials found widespread acceptance [5, 17]. The first synthetic graft material that was more widely accepted was polytetrafluoroethylene (PTFE), the chemical constituent of Teflon. Vascular surgery has been using this graft material for decades. In animal experiments, this material was well-tolerated; however, migration of the graft at the bladder anastomosis, as well as infection, hindered the success of PTFE [18, 19]. The porous form of PTFE, GoreTex (W. L. Gore & Associates, Inc., AZ, USA) was pursued further for use in ureteral reconstruction but remained limited to animal experiments. One shortcoming of this material was its tendency to lead to anastomotic strictures, which in part may be due to the lack of an urothelial lining [20, 21]. This lining can be derived from pre-seeded grafts (see below) or from in-growth of urothelial cells from the anastomotic ends. One important prerequisite of any graft material for ureteral substitution is that it must ensure a resilient ureteral lining with a dependable vascular supply. Without a reliable vascular network to supply nutrients, the luminal epithelium will not survive in the urinary tract.[19] Therefore, a successful graft will have to consist of a scaffold material that allows the in-growth of blood vessels and sustain a layer of seeded cells as well as growing urothelium from the anastomotic ends.

Ureteral graft requirements led to the development of semi-synthetic grafts in which modified xenograft material was used. Small intestinal submucosa (SIS) for example, has been employed in several animal studies with encouraging results as an urothelial lining formed in layers, recapitulating the native ureter [22-25]. This generated within 4 weeks in rabbits and pigs and obstruction was not observed. However, longer ureteral defects appear to be less amenable to successful repair with SIS as occlusion of the graft with resultant obstruction was observed [26, 27]. This is likely due to the inflammatory response causing a dense fibrotic growth, which in tubular grafts, leads to partial or complete obstruction [28]. Halifuginon, a collagen inhibitor, was used in attempts to prevent obstruction with lackluster results [26]. El-Hakim published a report in 2005 that described the use of de-epithelialized bowel autotransplantation in a Monti fashion that was seeded with cultured autologous urothelial cells which was then interposed in dog ureters [29]. No contraction, fibrosis, nor scar formation was observed and the ureters remained patent. However, intestinal mucosa regenerated underneath the urothelial lining at the anastomotic sites [29]. This study is notable for its attempt to generate grafts that use a scaffold seeded with urothelial cells although the scaffold material was not ideal. However, this study demonstrated the utility of an engineered graft consisting of a seeded scaffold.

Development and discoveries in material sciences allowed for the development of additional substances that have properties that make them novel candidates for the engineering of ureter grafts. One such material is a nanoporous scaffold made out of polycaprolactone-lecithin electrospun fibers. Such scaffolds are biocompatible and biodegradable like SIS yet easier to employ due to their mechanical properties. SIS is rather friable, especially when seeded, which makes tubularization very difficult. In contrast, polycaprolactone-lecithin electrospun fiber scaffolds can rather easily be formed into a tube structure prior to implantation [29]. The nanofibrous property that is achieved in the electrospinning process mimics the fibrous structure of extra-cellular matrix (ECM) in native ureters and provides an optimized environment to promote cellular growth and differentiation. The coating of these scaffolds with phospholipid lecithin provides cellular affinity for attachment and proliferation of urothelial cells, which in turn preserves both the transport and barrier functions of the urinary tract [30].

Advances in stem cell research and their regulation have also led to the employment of human stem cells in urologic research. Bone marrow-derived multipotent stem cells promote and accelerate angiogenesis by promoting endothelial differentiation, recruiting endogenous progenitor cells, and secreting a variety of growth factors [31, 32]. Stem cells also reduce inflammation and fibrosis, and have the ability to differentiate to replace damaged cells.[31] After co-culture with urothelium or urothelium-derived conditioned medium, multipotent stem cells exhibit an urothelial phenotype, expressing urothelium-specific genes and proteins [33, 34]. Recent tissue recombination model cells were able to undergo directed differentiation toward endodermal-derived urothelium and development into mature bladder tissue [35]. Hence, stem cell-seeded scaffolds have been employed successfully for bladder reconstruction; one report also describes their use for ureteral reconstruction [36]. Liao et al describe a ureteral graft on the basis of acellular bladder matrix seeded with bone marrow-derived stem cells [37]. Briefly, acellular bladder matrix was made from a harvested rabbit bladder that was digested with collagenases, proteases, and nucleases to ensure that only a scaffold of fibers and matrix remained. Multipotent bone-marrow derived stem cells were then seeded on both sides of the matrix. After in vitro culturing for several days, a tubular structure around a catheter was formed. This tubularized graft was then implanted into the omentum of rabbits to facilitate angiogenesis and vascularization. Two weeks later, the vascularized graft was used to bridge a 4 cm long defect of one ureter and connected proximally and distally with end-to-end anastomoses to the ureter. An urothelial lining with muscle fibers was present after 4, 8 and 16 weeks; multilayer urothelium covered the entire lumen with central visible neovascularization and organized smooth muscle bundles. [37] One drawback of this study is limited translation from animal to human model. Although this material exhibits properties that make it a suitable carrier substance for stem cells, it not only requires an additional operation to harvest a bladder segment, it also demands a sufficiently large segment of bladder tissue which undoubtedly will impact bladder capacity and function. Another option would be generation of acellular bladder matrix from cadaveric specimens, which will come at the expense of organ shortage, potential for disease initiation and progression, and ethical hurdles. Immunosuppression may also be required. Animal acellular bladder grafts can be considered as well. It remains questionable whether the incubation of the initial seeded graft in omentum may be omitted by the use of another fully synthetic scaffold, which would spare the patient the operation of omental harvesting.

Several studies have addressed the use of tissue-engineered grafts in humans in other urologic organs. Atala et al have employed tissue-engineered cystoplasty grafts in three bladders of patients with myelomeningoceles associated with end-stage bladder disease.[38] The grafts were engineered from polyglycolic acid, a material commonly used for hernia repairs, to serve as a scaffold for cultured urothelial and muscle cells obtained from a bladder biopsy [38]. A similar graft was recently described for the reconstruction of human urethras [39]. In this study a modified polyglycolic acid-based material (polyglycolic acid:poly (lactide-co- glycolide acid)) was seeded with urothelial and smooth muscle cells and used for the generation of a tubularized graft which was employed to bridge defects in the urethra of 4-6 cm in length. The grafts showed a histologically accurate urethral architecture by 3 months, demonstrating distinguishable layers of epithelia and smooth muscle; all grafts remained patent after a mean follow-up of nearly 6 years [39]. Both studies confirmed that synthetic graft employment for urologic reconstruction is possible. Furthermore, they proved that stem cells obtained from a biopsy were sufficient for supplying the mucosal lining and obtaining sufficient vascularization without prior omental incubation of the graft.

Outlook for the Future

As demonstrated for bladder and urethra, tissue-engineered grafts are showing very promising results when used in a clinical setting. [38, 39] Concerns about calculus formation, permeability to urine, bio-incompatibility or strictures should therefore not prevent urologists from using tissue-engineered grafts for ureteral reconstruction and replacement. The next step in the development of ureteral grafts will be to translate those tissue-engineered graft animal models to clinical trials. Technology is undoubtedly sufficiently advanced to produce grafts that are capable of sufficient vascularization and bear an inner urothelial lining [38, 39]. Stem cell impregnated scaffolds with its associated angiogenesis may be especially helpful for mid ureteral replacement as the vascular supply here is sparse. Although bone marrow aspiration for stem cell harvest is slightly more invasive than cystoscopy and biopsy, the additional benefit of having a multi-potent cell capable of differentiating into a multi-layered ureteral graft that alleviates the co-culturing of several cell types such as urothelium and muscle, warrant this approach. For reconstruction of shorter ureteral defects, incubation in omentum prior to use for substitution may not be necessary if care is taken to preserve vascular supply during ureter dissection, especially at the anastomotic ends. Clinical studies will have to further analyze this. Ideally, a randomized controlled study would compare tissue-engineered grafts with ileal ureters, but in light of the overall small case numbers, this may not be possible to do.

Conclusion

Surgical techniques for ureteral reconstruction and replacement have been unchanged for over half a century. Though there may be only little room for improvement in techniques for the reconstruction of small ureteral defects, ureteral substitution for larger defects can make vast improvements since current substitution is dependent on bowel segments with considerable associated drawbacks. Success rates with ileal ureters are acceptable, but complications do occur. Attempts to substitute the ureter with several synthetic materials over the past 30 years have failed. Recent technological advances have provided biologically inert scaffold materials that encourage vascular ingrowth and mucosal re-epithelialization. The ideal cell type for seeding appears to be bone marrow-derived multipotent stem cells because of their strong angiogenic properties and ability to differentiate into multiple cell types to best mimic the layers of the native ureter. Engineered urologic tissue consisting of cell-seeded scaffolds has been successfully employed for the reconstruction of human bladders and urethras. It will be the future of ureteral reconstruction.

References

[1]   Siram, S. M., Gerald, S. Z., Greene, W. R. et al.: Ureteral trauma: patterns and mechanisms of injury of an uncommon condition. *Am J Surg,* 199: 566, 2010.

[2]   Abboudi, H., Ahmed, K., Royle, J. et al.: Ureteric injury: a challenging condition to diagnose and manage. *Nat Rev Urol,* 10: 108, 2012.

[3]   Parpala-Sparman, T., Paananen, I., Santala, M. et al.: Increasing numbers of ureteric injuries after the introduction of laparoscopic surgery. *Scand J Urol Nephrol,* 42: 422, 2008.

[4]   Iwaszko, M. R., Krambeck, A. E., Chow, G. K. et al.: Transureteroureterostomy revisited: long-term surgical outcomes. *J Urol,* 183: 1055, 2010.

[5]   Wagenknecht, L. V., Auvert, J.: [Substitution of the human ureter using synthetic material]. *Chirurg*, 43: 334, 1972.

[6]   Pope, J., Koch, M. O.: Ureteral replacement with reconfigured colon substitute. *J Urol,* 155: 1693, 1996.

[7]   Obaidah, A., Mane, S. B., Dhende, N. P. et al.: Our experience of ureteral substitution in pediatric age group. *Urology*, 75: 1476, 2010.

[8]   Springer, A., Reck, C. A., Fartacek, R. et al.: Appendix vermiformis as a left pyelo-ureteral substitute in a 6-month-old girl with solitary kidney. *Afr J Paediatr Surg*, 8: 218, 2011.

[9]   Rack, F. J.: Ureteroileal neocystostomy; use of ileal segment as substitute ureter; report of a case. *J Am Med Assoc*, 152: 516, 1953.

[10]   Tveter, K. J., Bloom, D. A., Goodwin, W. E.: Ileal ureter: current status. *Eur Urol*, 6: 321, 1980.

[11]   Armatys, S. A., Mellon, M. J., Beck, S. D. et al.: Use of ileum as ureteral replacement in urological reconstruction. *J Urol,* 181: 177, 2009.

[12]   Chung, B. I., Hamawy, K. J., Zinman, L. N. et al.: The use of bowel for ureteral replacement for complex ureteral reconstruction: long-term results. *J Urol,* 175: 179, 2006.

[13]   Matlaga, B. R., Shah, O. D., Hart, L. J. et al.: Ileal ureter substitution: a contemporary series. *Urology*, 62: 998, 2003.

[14]   Lubash, S.: Experiences with tantalum tubes in the reimplantation of the ureters into the sigmoid in dogs and humans. *J Urol*, 57: 1010, 1947.

[15]   Ulm, A. H.: Total replacement of the human ureter with teflon prosthesis. *J Urol*, 96: 455, 1966.

[16]   Hodge, A. D.: Teflon replacement of the ureter. *N Z Med J,* 62: 39, 1963.

[17]   Wagenknecht, L. V., Auvert, J., Sausse, A.: Ureteral replacement with synthetic prothesis in dogs. *Eur Surg Res*, 4: 131, 1972.

[18]   Dreikorn, K., Lobelenz, J., Horsch, R. et al.: Alloplastic replacement of the canine ureter by expanded polytetrafluoroethylene (gore-tex) grafts. Preliminary report. *Eur Urol*, 4: 379, 1978.

[19]   Varady, S., Friedman, E., Yap, W. T. et al.: Ureteral replacement with a new synthetic material: Gore-Tex. *J Urol*, 128: 171, 1982.

[20]   Baltaci, S., Ozer, G., Ozer, E. et al.: Failure of ureteral replacement with Gore-Tex tube grafts. *Urology*, 51: 400, 1998.

[21]   Sabanegh, E. S., Jr., Downey, J. R., Sago, A. L.: Long-segment ureteral replacement with expanded polytetrafluoroethylene grafts. *Urology*, 48: 312, 1996.

[22] Jaffe, J. S., Ginsberg, P. C., Yanoshak, S. J. et al.: Ureteral segment replacement using a circumferential small-intestinal submucosa xenogenic graft. *J Invest Surg*, 14: 259, 2001.

[23] Liatsikos, E. N., Dinlenc, C. Z., Kapoor, R. et al.: Laparoscopic ureteral reconstruction with small intestinal submucosa. *J Endourol*, 15: 217, 2001.

[24] Xie, H., Shaffer, B. S., Wadia, Y. et al.: Use of reconstructed small intestine submucosa for urinary tract replacement. *ASAIO J*, 46: 268, 2000.

[25] Smith, T. G., 3rd, Gettman, M., Lindberg, G. et al.: Ureteral replacement using porcine small intestine submucosa in a porcine model. *Urology*, 60: 931, 2002.

[26] Duchene, D. A., Jacomides, L., Ogan, K. et al.: Ureteral replacement using small-intestinal submucosa and a collagen inhibitor in a porcine model. *J Endourol*, 18: 507, 2004.

[27] El-Assmy, A., Hafez, A. T., El-Sherbiny, M. T. et al.: Use of single layer small intestinal submucosa for long segment ureteral replacement: a pilot study. *J Urol,* 171: 1939, 2004.

[28] Sofer, M., Rowe, E., Forder, D. M. et al.: Ureteral segmental replacement using multilayer porcine small-intestinal submucosa. *J Endourol*, 16: 27, 2002.

[29] El-Hakim, A., Marcovich, R., Chiu, K. Y. et al.: First prize: ureteral segmental replacement revisited. *J Endourol*, 19: 1069, 2005.

[30] Shen, J., Fu, X., Ou, L. et al.: Construction of ureteral grafts by seeding urothelial cells and bone marrow mesenchymal stem cells into polycaprolactone-lecithin electrospun fibers. *Int J Artif Organs*, 33: 161, 2010.

[31] Vaegler, M., Lenis, A. T., Daum, L. et al.: Stem cell therapy for voiding and erectile dysfunction. *Nat Rev Urol*, 2012.

[32] Kaigler, D., Krebsbach, P. H., Polverini, P. J. et al.: Role of vascular endothelial growth factor in bone marrow stromal cell modulation of endothelial cells. *Tissue Eng*, 9: 95, 2003.

[33] Tian, H., Bharadwaj, S., Liu, Y. et al.: Myogenic differentiation of human bone marrow mesenchymal stem cells on a 3D nano fibrous scaffold for bladder tissue engineering. *Biomaterials*, 31: 870, 2010.

[34] Tian, H., Bharadwaj, S., Liu, Y. et al.: Differentiation of human bone marrow mesenchymal stem cells into bladder cells: potential for urological tissue engineering. *Tissue Eng Part A*, 16: 1769, 2010.

[35] Anumanthan, G., Makari, J. H., Honea, L. et al.: Directed differentiation of bone marrow derived mesenchymal stem cells into bladder urothelium. *J Urol,* 180: 1778, 2008.

[36] Sharma, A. K., Bury, M. I., Fuller, N. J. et al.: Cotransplantation with specific populations of spina bifida bone marrow stem/progenitor cells enhances urinary bladder regeneration. *Proc Natl Acad Sci U S A*, 110: 4003, 2013.

[37] Liao, W., Yang, S., Song, C. et al.: Construction of ureteral grafts by seeding bone marrow mesenchymal stem cells and smooth muscle cells into bladder acellular matrix. Transplant Proc, 45: 730, 2013.

[38] Atala, A., Bauer, S. B., Soker, S. et al.: Tissue-engineered autologous bladders for patients needing cystoplasty. *Lancet*, 367: 1241, 2006.

[39] Raya-Rivera, A., Esquiliano, D. R., Yoo, J. J. et al.: Tissue-engineered autologous urethras for patients who need reconstruction: an observational study. *Lancet*, 377: 1175, 2011.

Index

U

V

W

Y